Editors

ASIF M. ILYAS
SAQIB REHMAN
GILES R. SCUDERI
FELASFA M. WODAJO

ORTHOPEDIC CLINICS OF NORTH AMERICA

www.orthopedic.theclinics.com

April 2014 • Volume 45 • Number 2

ELSEVIER

1600 John F. Kennedy Boulevard • Suite 1800 • Philadelphia, Pennsylvania, 19103-2899.

http://www.orthopedic.theclinics.com

ORTHOPEDIC CLINICS OF NORTH AMERICA Volume 45, Number 2
April 2014 ISSN 0030-5898, ISBN-13: 978-0-323-29481-2

Editor: Jennifer Flynn-Briggs
Developmental Editor: Stephanie Carter

Orthopedic Clinics of North America (ISSN 0030-5898) is published quarterly by Elsevier Inc., 360 Park Avenue South, New York, NY 10010-1710. Months of issue are January, April, July, and October. Business and Editorial Offices: 1600 John F. Kennedy Blvd., Suite 1800, Philadelphia, PA 19103-2899. Customer Service Office: 3251 Riverport Lane, Maryland Heights, MO 63043. Periodicals postage paid at New York, NY and additional mailing offices. Subscription prices are $310.00 per year for (US individuals), $596.00 per year for (US institutions), $365.00 per year (Canadian individuals), $727.00 per year (Canadian institutions), $450.00 per year (international individuals), $727.00 per year (international institutions), $150.00 per year (US students), $220.00 per year (Canadian and international students). Foreign air speed delivery is included in all *Clinics* subscription prices. All prices are subject to change without notice. **POSTMASTER:** Send change of address to *Orthopedic Clinics of North America*, **Elsevier Health Sciences Division, Subscription Customer Service, 3251 Riverport Lane, Maryland Heights, MO 63043. Customer Service (orders, claims, online, change of address): Elsevier Health Sciences Division, Subscription Customer Service, 3251 Riverport Lane, Maryland Heights, MO 63043. Tel: 1-800-654-2452 (U.S. and Canada); 314-447-8871 (outside U.S. and Canada). Fax: 314-447-8029. E-mail: journalscustomerservice-usa@elsevier. com (for print support); journalsonlinesupport-usa@elsevier.com (for online support).**

Reprints. For copies of 100 or more, of articles in this publication, please contact the Commercial Reprints Department, Elsevier Inc., 360 Park Avenue South, New York, NY 10010-1710. Tel.: 212-633-3874; Fax: 212-633-3820; E-mail: reprints@elsevier. com.

Orthopedic Clinics of North America is covered in *MEDLINE/PubMed* (*Index Medicus*), *Cinahl, Excerpta Medica,* and *Cumulative Index to Nursing and Allied Health Literature.*

Printed and bound by CPI Group (UK) Ltd, Croydon, CR0 4YY

Contributors

EDITORS

ASIF M. ILYAS, MD - *Upper Extremity*
Program Fellowship Director of Hand and
Upper Extremity Surgery, Rothman Institute
Associate Professor of Orthopaedic Surgery,
Thomas Jefferson University, Philadelphia,
Pennsylvania

SAQIB REHMAN, MD - *Trauma*
Director of Orthopaedic Trauma, Associate
Professor of Orthopaedic Surgery, Temple
University Hospital, Philadelphia, Pennsylvania

GILES R. SCUDERI, MD - *Adult
Reconstruction*
Vice President, Orthopedic Service Line,
Northshore LIJ Health System; Director, ISK
Institute, New York, New York

FELASFA M. WODAJO, MD - *Oncology*
Musculoskeletal Tumor Surgery, Virginia
Hospital Center, Arlington, Virginia

AUTHORS

JOSHUA M. ABZUG, MD
Assistant Professor, Department of
Orthopedics, Director, University of Maryland
Brachial Plexus Clinic, University of Maryland
School of Medicine, Timonium, Maryland

JOSE I. ALBERGO, MD
Orthopaedic Oncology Service, Department of
Orthopedics, Italian Hospital of Buenos Aires,
Buenos Aires, Argentina

LOUIS-PHILIPPE AMIOT, MD, MSc
Zimmer CAS, Montreal, Canada

JACK ANAVIAN, MD
Resident, Department of Orthopaedic Surgery,
Warren Alpert Medical School of Brown
University, Providence, Rhode Island

CHRISTOPHER ANDERSON, MS
Director of Clinical Research, Department of
Bioengineering and Clinical Research,
OrthoSensor Inc, Dania, Florida

LUIS A. APONTE-TINAO, MD
Orthopaedic Oncology Service, Department of
Orthopedics, Italian Hospital of Buenos Aires,
Buenos Aires, Argentina

MIGUEL A. AYERZA, MD
Orthopaedic Oncology Service, Department of
Orthopedics, Italian Hospital of Buenos Aires,
Buenos Aires, Argentina

MARIE-JOSEE BERTHIAUME, MD
Hopital Maisonneuve-Rosemont, Montreal,
Canada

CHRISTOPHER BOONE, MD
Private Pratice, Department of Orthopaedics,
Tacoma, Washington, USA

DAVID A. CAMARATA, MD, FAAOS
Ortho Arizona: Arizona Bone and Joint
Specialists, Scottsdale, Arizona

JASKARNDIP CHAHAL, MD, FRCSC
Sports Medicine Program, Division of
Orthopaedic Surgery, Department of
Surgery, Women's College Hospital,
University of Toronto, Toronto, Ontario,
Canada

BRIAN J. COLE, MD, MBA
Professor, Division of Sports Medicine,
Midwest Orthopaedics at Rush, Chicago,
Illinois

MATTHEW W. COLMAN, MD
Department of Orthopedic Surgery, Boston
Children's Hospital, Beth Israel Deaconess
Hospital, Massachusetts General Hospital,
Boston, Massachusetts

DANIEL DEBOTTIS, MD
Fellow, Division of Shoulder and Elbow
Surgery, Department of Orthopaedic Surgery,
Warren Alpert Medical School of Brown
University, Providence, Rhode Island

LEAH ELSON, BSc
Researcher, Department of Bioengineering and
Clinical Research, OrthoSensor Inc, Dania,
Florida

MICHEL FALLAHA, MD
Hopital Maisonneuve-Rosemont, Montreal,
Canada

GERMAN L. FARFALLI, MD
Orthopaedic Oncology Service, Department of
Orthopedics, Italian Hospital of Buenos Aires,
Buenos Aires, Argentina

JONATHAN M. FRANK, MD
Resident Physician, Department of
Orthopaedic Surgery, Rush University
Medical Center, Chicago, Illinois

RACHEL M. FRANK, MD
Resident Physician, Department of
Orthopaedic Surgery, Rush University
Medical Center, Chicago, Illinois

MARK GEBHARDT, MD
Department of Orthopedic Surgery, Boston
Children's Hospital, Beth Israel Deaconess
Hospital, Boston, Massachusetts

MICHAEL GITHENS, MD
Resident, Department of Orthopaedic Surgery,
Stanford University School of Medicine,
Stanford, California

ANDREW GREEN, MD
Associate Professor and Chief, Division of
Shoulder and Elbow Surgery, Department of
Orthopaedic Surgery, Warren Alpert Medical
School of Brown University, Providence,
Rhode Island

CHRISTINA J. GUTOWSKI, MD, MPH
Department of Orthopaedic Surgery, Thomas
Jefferson University Hospital, Philadelphia,
Pennsylvania

FRANCIS J. HORNICEK, MD, PhD
Department of Orthopedic Surgery,
Massachusetts General Hospital, Boston,
Massachusetts

ASIF M. ILYAS, MD
Program Fellowship Director of Hand and
Upper Extremity Surgery, Rothman Institute
Associate Professor of Orthopaedic Surgery,
Thomas Jefferson University, Philadelphia,
Pennsylvania

SCOTT H. KOZIN, MD
Clinical Professor, Department of Orthopaedic
Surgery, Chief of Staff, Shriners Hospitals for
Children, Temple University, Philadelphia,
Pennsylvania

PATRICK LAVIGNE, MD, PhD
Hopital Maisonneuve-Rosemont, Montreal,
Canada

DAVID W. LOWENBERG, MD
Clinical Professor, Chief, Orthopaedic Trauma
Service, Department of Orthopaedic Surgery,
Stanford University School of Medicine,
Stanford, California

SANTIAGO LOZANO-CALDERON, MD, PhD
Department of Orthopedic Surgery, Boston
Children's Hospital, Beth Israel Deaconess
Hospital, Massachusetts General Hospital,
Boston, Massachusetts

VINCENT MASSE, MD
Hopital Maisonneuve-Rosemont, Montreal,
Canada

DAVID MAYMAN, BA, MD
Assistant Professor, Assistant Attending,
Orthopedic Surgery, Hospital for Special
Surgery, Cornell University, New York,
New York

D. LUIS MUSCOLO, MD
Orthopaedic Oncology Service, Department of
Orthopedics, Italian Hospital of Buenos Aires,
Buenos Aires, Argentina

KEVIN A. RASKIN, MD
Department of Orthopedic Surgery,
Massachusetts General Hospital, Boston,
Massachusetts

LUCAS E. RITACCO, MD
Department of Orthopedics, Italian Hospital of Buenos Aires; Virtual Planning and Navigation Unit, Department of Health Informatics, Italian Hospital of Buenos Aires, Buenos Aires, Argentina

MARTIN ROCHE, MD
Chief of Orthopedics, Holy Cross Hospital, Orthopaedic Institute, Fort Lauderdale, Florida

ANTHONY A. ROMEO, MD
Professor, Division of Sports Medicine, Midwest Orthopaedics at Rush, Chicago, Illinois

GILES R. SCUDERI, MD
Vice President, Orthopedic Service Line, Northshore LIJ Health System; Director, ISK Institute, New York, New York

NIKHIL N. VERMA, MD
Assistant Professor, Division of Sports Medicine, Midwest Orthopaedics at Rush, Chicago, Illinois

Contributors

LUCAS E. RITACCO, MD
Department of Orthopaedics, Italian Hospital of Buenos Aires; Virtual Planning and Navigation Unit, Department of Health Informatics, Italian Hospital of Buenos Aires, Buenos Aires, Argentina

MARTIN ROCHE, MD
Chief of Orthopedics, Holy Cross Hospital, Orthopaedic Institute, Fort Lauderdale, Florida

ANTHONY A. ROMEO, MD
Professor, Division of Sports Medicine, Midwest Orthopaedics at Rush, Chicago, Illinois

GILES R. SCUDERI, MD
Vice President, Orthopedic Service Line, Northshore LIJ Health System; Director, ISK Institute, New York, New York

NIKHIL N. VERMA, MD
Assistant Professor, Division of Sports Medicine, Midwest Orthopaedics at Rush, Chicago, Illinois

Contents

Adult Reconstruction

Achieving optimal soft tissue balance intraoperatively is a critical element for a successful outcome after total knee arthroplasty. Although advances in navigation have improved the incidence of angular outliers, spatial distance measurements do not quantify soft tissue stability or degrees of ligament tension. Revisions caused by instability, malrotation, and malalignment still constitute up to one-third of early knee revisions. The development of integrated microelectronics and sensors into the knee trials during surgery allows surgeons to evaluate and act on real-time data regarding implant position, rotation, alignment, and soft tissue balance through a full range of motion.

Total knee arthroplasty is a common procedure, and current navigation systems are gradually gaining acceptance for improving surgical accuracy and clinical outcomes. A new navigation system used within the surgical field, iAssist, has demonstrated reproducible accuracy in component alignment. All orientation information is captured by small electronic pods and transmitted via a local wireless network, which directs the surgical workflow automatically to the femoral and tibial resection instruments. This simple and accurate navigation system used completely in the surgical field, without optical trackers or preoperative imaging, seems to be the latest generation of smart instrumentation for total knee arthroplasty.

This article presents a concise description and literature review of the eLibra Dynamic Ligament Balancing Device in total knee arthroplasty. This device is a force sensor that allows surgeons to balance the medial and lateral collateral ligaments during total knee replacement. This instrument provides precise, quantitative, digital information in newtons during surgery that allows surgeons to accurately externally rotate the femoral component in order to balance the forces across the medial and lateral compartments. The device is highly accurate and simple to use. It relies on objective dynamic data to balance the knee rather than static landmarks or subjective tensiometers.

Computer navigation for knee replacement surgery has been available for over a decade but has not gained popularity despite improved accuracy. The literature has shown higher failure rates for knee replacements with tibial malalignment. This article reviews some of this literature and demonstrates a novel handheld, simple-to-use, disposable navigation system that has been proven to be accurate and may be the answer to combining ease of use, lower cost, and increased accuracy to give better overall results.

Trauma

There is a growing mass of literature to suggest that circular external fixation for high-energy tibial fractures has advantages over traditional internal fixation, with potential improved rates of union, decreased incidence of posttraumatic osteomyelitis, and decreased soft tissue problems. To further advance our understanding of the role of circular external fixation in the management of these tibial fractures, randomized controlled trials should be implemented. In addition to complication rates and radiographic outcomes, validated functional outcome tools and cost analysis of this method should be compared with open reduction with internal fixation.

Because the greater tuberosity is the insertion site of the posterior superior rotator cuff, fractures can have a substantial impact on functional outcome. Isolated fractures should not inadvertently be trivialized. Thorough patient evaluation is required to make an appropriate treatment decision. In most cases surgical management is considered when there is displacement of 5 mm or greater. Although reduction of displaced greater tuberosity fractures has traditionally been performed with open techniques, arthroscopic techniques are now available. The most reliable techniques of fixation of the greater tuberosity incorporate the rotator cuff tendon bone junction rather than direct bone-to-bone fixation.

Upper Extremity

Acromioplasty is a well-described technique used throughout the wide spectrum of treatment options for shoulder impingement and rotator cuff pathology. Several randomized prospective studies have described clinical outcomes that are statistically similar when comparing patients undergoing rotator cuff repair either with or without concomitant acromioplasty. This article reviews the current evidence for use of acromioplasty in patients with subacromial impingement syndrome and during arthroscopic rotator cuff repair. Despite recently published studies, more long-term

data, especially with regard to failure rates and return-to-surgery rates over time, are
needed to better determine the role of acromioplasty.

Joshua M. Abzug and Scott H. Kozin

Brachial plexus birth palsy can result in permanent lifelong deficits and unfortunately
continues to be relatively common despite advancements in obstetric care. The
diagnosis can be made shortly after birth by physical examination, noting a lack of
movement in the affected upper extremity. Treatment begins with passive range-of-
motion exercises to maintain flexibility and tactile stimulation to provide sensory
reeducation. Primary surgery consists of microsurgical nerve surgery, whereas secondary surgery consists of alternative microsurgical procedures, tendon transfers,
or osteotomies, all of which improve outcomes in the short term. However, the
long-term outcomes of current treatment recommendations remain unknown.

Christina J. Gutowski and Asif M. Ilyas

Osteoporosis continues to be a major health condition plaguing the aging population. The major manifestation of osteoporosis, the development of fragility fractures, is a burden both clinically and economically on patients and the nation's
health care system, with up to half of all American women sustaining a fragility
fracture in their older years. The high frequency of injuries to the distal radius
and proximal humerus should lead upper extremity surgeons to take pause and
recognize the magnitude of impact these fractures have on their patient population.
Recommended interventions span a spectrum of aggressiveness and have various
financial implications.

Oncology

Felasfa M. Wodajo

Matthew W. Colman, Santiago Lozano-Calderon, Kevin A. Raskin, Francis J. Hornicek,
and Mark Gebhardt

Non-neoplastic soft tissue masses may mimic soft tissue sarcoma in a wide variety
of clinical settings. Systematic and thorough review of patient history, physical examination, imaging, laboratory results, and biopsy will allow the clinician to differentiate between the two in most cases. We describe several common non-neoplastic
entities that may mimic soft tissue sarcoma in case presentation format along with
the characteristics that help distinguish them.

Luis A. Aponte-Tinao, Lucas E. Ritacco, Jose I. Albergo, Miguel A. Ayerza, D. Luis Muscolo,
and German L. Farfalli

 Videos of fresh frozen allografts in bone and joint reconstruction accompany
this article

Fresh frozen allograft reconstruction has been used for a long time in massive bone
loss in orthopedic surgery. Allografts have the advantage of being biologic

reconstructions, which gives them durability. Despite a greater number of complications in the short term, after 5 years these stabilize with high rates of survival after 10 years. The rate of early complications and the need for careful management in the first years has led the orthopedic surgeon to the use of other options. However, the potential durability of this reconstruction makes this one of the best options for younger patients with high life expectancy.

ORTHOPEDIC CLINICS OF NORTH AMERICA

FORTHCOMING ISSUES

Beginning with the July 2013 issue, *Orthopedic Clinics of North America* began to appear in this new format. Rather than focusing on a single topic, each issue contains articles on key areas in orthopedics—adult reconstruction, upper extremity, trauma, pediatrics and oncology. Articles on sports medicine and foot and ankle will also be included on a regular basis. As the practice of orthopedics has become more specialized, the format of one topic per issue is no longer fulfilling our readers' needs. The new format is intended to address these changing needs.

Orthopedic Clinics of North America continues to publish a print issue four times a year, in January, April, July, and October. However, this series also includes online-only articles that will be published on a rolling basis (not in accordance with our quarterly publication dates). These articles, along with articles from our print issues, are available on http://www.orthopedic.theclinics.com/.

DOWNLOAD Free App!

Review Articles
THE CLINICS

YOUR iPhone and iPad

Adult Reconstruction

Preface
Adult Reconstruction

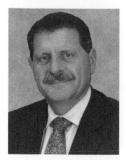

Giles R. Scuderi, MD
Editor

In the last decade, instrumentation for total knee arthroplasty has improved the accuracy, reproducibility, and reliability of the procedure. The introduction of computer navigation moved surgeons into the arena of advanced technology and leads us into the development of improved medical imaging, sensor technology, and interactive enabling instrumentation, which further optimize the accuracy of surgery. The successful use of these intelligent technologies requires that it supports the surgeon with enhanced feedback, integrates the intraoperative information into the surgical workflow, and provides visual dexterity while performing the procedure. Soft tissue balancing is important in the outcome of total knee arthroplasty, and force sensor technology allows for intra-operative dynamic balancing of the supporting ligaments with fine-tuning and real-time feedback. This has the potential to translate the intraoperative qualitative feel of a balanced knee into a quantitative measurement that is accurate and reproducible. The results of total knee arthroplasty also benefit from the accuracy of knee alignment, relying on the bone resection with proper positioning of components. Incorporating intelligence into the resection guides with gyroscopes and accelerometers provides reproducible accuracy without the complexity of image-guided navigation systems. This current issue of *Orthopedic Clinics of North America* covers some of the most recent technologic advances in total knee arthroplasty and describes some of the smart technologies that help facilitate the procedure.

Giles R. Scuderi, MD
Orthopedic Service Line
Northshore LIJ Health System
New York, NY, USA

ISK Institute
New York, NY, USA

E-mail address:
grscuderi@nshs.edu

Orthop Clin N Am 45 (2014) xiii
http://dx.doi.org/10.1016/j.ocl.2014.01.002
0030-5898/14/$ – see front matter © 2014 Elsevier Inc. All rights reserved.

Dynamic Soft Tissue Balancing in Total Knee Arthroplasty

Martin Roche, MD[a], Leah Elson, BSc[b], Christopher Anderson, MS[b],*

KEYWORDS

- Total knee arthroplasty • Sensor • Soft-tissue balancing • Smart tibial trials • Dynamic balancing
- Balancing verification

KEY POINTS

- Historically, ligamentous tension and laxity have not been measured and thus have not been quantified to correlate with patient outcomes.
- Intraoperative sensors can guide and confirm correction of soft tissue imbalance.
- Intraoperative sensors can communicate the effects of implant alignment and rotation on soft tissue balance.
- Intraoperative sensors allow the evaluation of the effects of implant kinematic design on the kinetic profile of the knee joint.

LIGAMENTOUS IMBALANCE AND INCIDENCE OF REVISION

A successful total knee arthroplasty can alleviate pain and reestablish proper kinetics to an arthritic joint.[1-3] This highly effective procedure is performed in more than 500,000 new patients in the United States every year, and this number is expected to reach 3.48 million by 2030.[4]

Although the survivorship of total knee arthroplasty components is greater than 90% at 15 years, the revision burden (defined as the ratio of revision to the total number of arthroplasties) has not improved for the past decade.[5-7]

The clinical and economic implications for revision surgery are underappreciated. More than 55,000 revision surgeries were performed in 2010 in the United States, with 48% of these revisions performed in patients younger than 65 years. Total costs associated with each revision total knee arthroplasty have been estimated to exceed $49,000. The current annual economic burden of revision knee surgery is $2.7 billion in hospital charges alone. By 2030, assuming a 5-fold increase in the number of revision procedures, this economic burden will exceed $13 billion annually.[5]

The number of revision total knee arthroplasties is expected to continue to increase, in concert with the rapidly increasing number of primary procedures, over the next 20 years.[4] Thus, new technologies that limit the factors associated with an increased risk of revision are now paramount to both the continued success of primary total knee replacement and reducing the economic burden associated with revision procedures themselves.

Joint infection is still the foremost cause of early revision. However, instability, malrotation, malalignment, component loosening, and patellofemoral complications all result from surgical technique that inadequately addresses soft tissue balance.[6-9]

Instability is cited in up to 22% of reported reasons for revision.[7] In patients exhibiting instability, excessive laxity in the soft tissues can cause pain, effusions, and an inability to navigate curbs and inclined planes.[8]

Conflict of Interest Statement: M. Roche is a board member of OrthoSensor, Inc. L. Elson and C. Anderson are both paid employees of OrthoSensor, Inc.

a Holy Cross Hospital, Orthopaedic Institute, 5597 North Dixie Highway, Fort Lauderdale, FL 33334, USA;
b Department of Bioengineering and Clinical Research, OrthoSensor Inc, 1855 Griffin Road, Suite A-310, Dania Beach, FL 33004-2200, USA
* Corresponding author.
E-mail address: canderson@orthosensor.com

Component loosening (up to 17% of early-stage revision; 34% of late-stage revision) is often a secondary effect of accelerated polyethylene wear.[7] Polyethylene microdebris disseminates into the joint space and causes an inflammatory immune response.[10,11] This inflammation results in osteolysis and disintegration of the bone–component interface. Accelerated wear is seen in patients with excessive soft tissue tension medially, laterally, and in the flexion gap from an excessively tight posterior cruciate ligament (PCL).[10,12]

Malalignment and patellofemoral complications caused by maltracking can lead to anterior pain, patellar instability, patellar fracture, and tibiofemoral flexion instability. These complications can occur from tibiofemoral rotational incongruency, commonly caused by internal rotation of the tibial tray, femoral component, or both.[13,14]

Reduction in the occurrence of these soft tissue related complications is essential for minimizing the percentage of revision procedures after total knee arthroplasty. Real-time data, presented intraoperatively, can assist the surgeon in reducing surgical outliers and achieving a well-aligned and well-balanced knee.

DEFINING BALANCE
Traditional Methods for Defining Balance

To achieve gap balance, most surgeons typically use spacer blocks to confirm that the extension and flexion gaps of the joint are equal with respect to a fixed distance measurement. This gap measurement dictates composite thickness of the final implant.[15,16]

Surgeons then rely on tactile navigation with their own hands, assessing coronal plane balance through applying a varus-valgus moment to the joint and evaluating the relative opening in each compartment.

Spacer blocks provide information on joint gaps and the alignment of cuts, but are not sensitive to soft tissue balance in the sagittal plane. When using spacer blocks, defining coronal intercompartmental balance in mid flexion and full flexion is often inconsistent, secondary to the open capsule, a subluxed patella, and hip rotation.

Surgical approaches to prepare the knee joint for the final prosthesis vary based on surgeon training and instrumentation. The 2 standard methods that are well documented are

1. Measured resection: a technique in which the surgeon makes all bony cuts based on anatomic references, then uses the trial implants to balance soft tissue tension.

2. Gap balancing: a technique in which the extension gap is balanced after the distal femur and proximal tibia are resected. The flexion gap is then distracted at 90°, allowing ligament tension to guide the femoral rotation.

Several factors contribute to inaccuracy in restoring normal balance and alignment in total knee arthroplasty when using either of the previously mentioned techniques. First, bony landmarks currently used to determine femoral rotation have been shown to be inaccurate, particularly in a deformed arthritic knee.[2] Second, soft tissue releases do not always affect flexion and extension gap balance symmetrically.[14,17] Finally, optimizing tibiofemoral balance can sometimes negatively affect patellofemoral tracking.[18,19]

The difficulties in achieving balance persist despite the availability of the techniques described earlier, because determining the degree of ligament balance in total knee arthroplasty has traditionally been established by the subjective assessment of each surgeon. Surgical results achieved by these subjective methods have been variable without the availability of intraoperative data to correlate techniques to outcomes.[14,18–23] Until recently, no method was available with which to quantify the relative "feel" of a joint when guiding soft tissue release.

Novel Methods and a More Precise Definition of Balance

Technological advances in microelectronics have only recently made it possible for the surgeon to quantify how ligamenture surrounding the joint directly affects articular kinetics through a full range of motion. This new sensor-embedded technology allows the surgeon to adjust for soft tissue imbalance, while receiving dynamic visual feedback regarding the specific knee design, within each patient-specific soft tissue envelope. For the first time, subjective surgeon assessment can be quantified, and balance in the coronal and sagittal planes is verifiable.

The sensor-embedded microelectronic array is housed in the standard tibial insert (Fig. 1) trial to identify the effects of alignment, rotation, and ligamentous tension or laxity on the geometric design of the knee.

Clinical and biomechanical analyses have shown that optimal joint kinematics are best evaluated with the patella reduced and the medial capsule closed. The knee is taken through a full range of motion, and the intercompartmental load differential is examined in early flexion, mid flexion, and full flexion to detect coronal

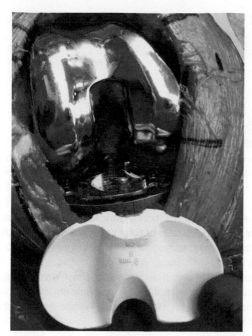

Fig. 1. Intraoperative knee showing replacement of the standard tibial trial with an "intelligent" trial.

plane asymmetry. The femoral rollback and posterior drawer is tested while the femoral contact points are evaluated to assess sagittal plane stability.

The development of sensor-embedded technology has allowed the construction and verification of a more scientifically based definition of *balance*. A new definition of *soft tissue gap* is exhibited from 10° to 110° of flexion. In terminal extension, the effects of compression, the screw-home mechanism, and the posterior capsule mask the effects of soft tissue tension or laxity (**Figs. 2–4**).

Therefore, the most useful application for this intraoperative data is to apply it to the evaluation of subtle joint imbalance, tibiofemoral rotational incongruency, and component malalignment.

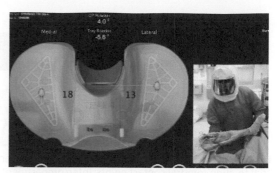

Fig. 3. Balanced loading at 10° flexion.

CLINICAL APPLICATIONS FOR DYNAMIC SOFT TISSUE BALANCING
Rotational Incongruency

Tibiofemoral rotational incongruency in total knee arthroplasty is associated with anterior knee pain, poor kinematic function, unfavorable patellar tracking, and decreased implant survivorship.[24] In one particular study, arrack and colleagues[13] showed that as little as 4.6° of internal rotation can cause anterior knee pain. Additionally, Berger and colleagues[14] reported that 5° to 8° of tibiofemoral rotational incongruency leads to patellar maltracking.

To establish an appropriate rotational orientation of the femoral component, anatomic reference points are commonly used.[13,19,25] Flexion distraction technique is also used to obtain a parallel flexion gap using the ligament tension in flexion to determine the femoral rotation.

When aligning the tibial tray, the mid to medial third of the tibial tubercle is commonly used. However, errors have been reported when using this landmark, because of a wide variance of up to 25° of rotation inherent in the line between tibial tubercle and posterior tibial plane.[26–29]

A retrospective analysis of intraoperative data from 100 consecutive total knee replacements found that 63.1% of patients exhibited an average of 6.3° ± 4.3° of asymmetrical tibiofemoral

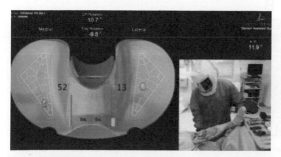

Fig. 2. Terminal extension with higher loads displayed on the medial side.

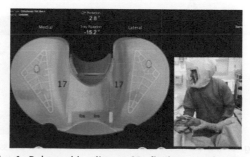

Fig. 4. Balanced loading at 90° flexion.

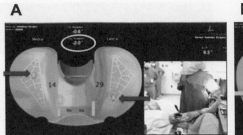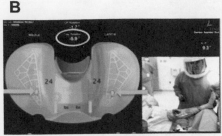

Fig. 5. (*A*) The knee is taken into extension and tibiofemoral incongruency is shown. (*B*) Surgeon adjusts the tibial trial to align femoral contact points; intercompartmental equalization of loads is achieved with correction of malrotation alone. The *arrows* are pointing out the location of femoral contact points on the tibial trial surface.

contact-point positioning in extension. Tibial tray rotation for all patients was initially dictated by the location of the mid-third of the tibial tubercle. Guided by intraoperative sensor feedback, the surgeon was able to correct all rotational incongruency in every case.[30]

Through incorporating intraoperative sensors, surgeons can set the rotation of the components using any method of their choosing. When the components are in place, any remaining tibiofemoral rotational incongruency can be corrected for using the location of femoral contact points, as shown dynamically on-screen by the sensor system.

With the placement of an anterior-medial or lateral pin to control for potential translation of the tray across the tibial plateau with trialing, the surgeon adjusts the tibial tray rotation until alignment of the femoral contact points is achieved (**Fig. 5**). These adjustments are evaluated and confirmed in real time. Central patellar tracking is then confirmed and the tray is pinned and stabilized. Optimal congruency is important to define before kinetic rollback and soft tissue balance are assessed. It is also seen that when the femoral condyles are relocated to the central tibial plateau and the femoral contact points are below 5° of rotation, soft tissue tension commonly equalizes. The belief is that this mechanism will improve anterior knee pain and stability through a full range of motion.

Appropriate rotational congruency is important for the survivorship of total knee arthroplasty components and, as suggested by literature, is difficult to attain.[26–29] Thus, advanced methods, such as using intraoperative sensors, may prove more useful than establishing references based on anatomic landmarks, which are inherently prone to variability.

Joint Imbalance

Coronal plane imbalance

During primary total knee arthroplasty, the surgeon may encounter excessive medial or lateral collateral ligament tension while addressing a varus or valgus knee. This excessive tension leads to increased loading in the medial or lateral compartment, which can be seen through a full range of motion. If uncorrected, the induced joint imbalance can culminate in unfavorable clinical outcomes, including pain, accelerated polyethylene degradation, joint instability, and limited range of motion.[10]

Although most surgeons can detect gross instability, judging ligament tension is difficult. However, the integration of intraoperative, sensor-embedded tibial inserts provides a way to evaluate tissue tension, and selectively optimize its release.

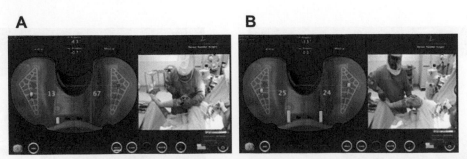

Fig. 6. (*A*) Surgeon identifies excessive medial pressure in mid flexion. (*B*) He selectively pie crusts the anterior bands of the medial collateral ligament to equalize loads in flexion, while avoiding anterior compartmental effects.

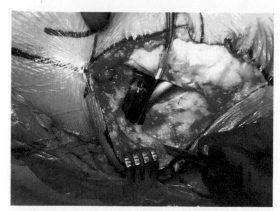

Fig. 7. Release of individual ligamentous fibers with an 18-gauge needle.

As part of an Institutional Review Board–approved multicentric evaluation, 232 patients were evaluated intraoperatively for joint imbalance (with *imbalance* defined as a mediolateral inter-compartmental loading difference of ≤15 lb). Using intraoperative-sensor feedback, soft tissue release was deemed necessary in 92.6% of patients to achieve balanced kinetics.[31]

Using the intraoperative sensors, surgeons can evaluate femoral contact point position and mediolateral intercompartmental loads (measured in pounds). Coronal asymmetric imbalance in flexion, mid flexion, and extension can now be recognized and defined. These data supplement any applied stress testing and allow the surgeon to close the medial capsule to identify the real soft tissue tension in flexion. If necessary, the surgeon can selectively titrate ligaments in a gradual fashion to avoid underreleasing or overreleasing (**Fig. 6**).

If medial or lateral imbalance is encountered, the surgeon may use the pie-crusting technique described by Bellemans and colleagues.[20] With this method, the surgeon first palpates the tissue to evaluate any fibers en tensio. Then, an 18-guage needle is used to sequentially pierce the structure of the ligament, perpendicularly to its fibrous growth pattern, releasing it to a balanced state (**Fig. 7**). This gradual release of fibers is tracked on-screen by the sensor system, and allows the surgeon to witness the dynamic change in load pressure.

Using a modified releasing technique, with real-time sensor data, the surgeon can release tension in the collateral ligamenture with quantified dynamic feedback. This gradual, digitally guided ligamentous release may prove to be a safer method than traditional transections, which may lead to underrelease or overrelease. Using a data-driven technique, the surgeon can confirm that both compartments of the bearing surface are loading proportionately in a selective approach.

Sagittal plane imbalance

Total knee arthroplasty components that incorporate a posterior substituting or cruciate retaining design have shown excellent long-term clinical results.[4] However, imbalance in the sagittal plane can still present with well-aligned implants. Although flexion instability may be seen more commonly in a PCL design, revision studies show that Posterior Stabilized (PS) designs can exhibit instability, especially in the posterior lateral corner during a flexion varus moment (ie, putting on shoes). Symmetric imbalance is typically seen with an overresected posterior femur, excessive tibial slope, or incompetent PCL, whereas an asymmetric imbalance is seen with improper femoral rotation or an overtensioned PCL.[32]

A balanced sagittal plane exhibits neither excessive tension nor laxity of the PCL. When taken into passive flexion, the femoral component undergoes symmetric rollback without anterior lift-off of the tibial insert (**Fig. 8**).

When evaluating flexion gap stability, it is imperative to reduce the patella and close the medial capsule to minimize error in assessing stability.

A posterior drawer test is applied at 90° of flexion and the femoral contact points are evaluated. In a

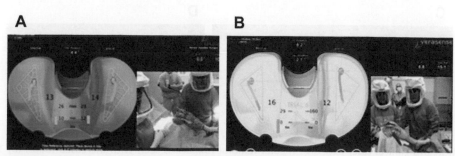

Fig. 8. The kinetic tracking feature allows assessment of femoral rollback (*A*) and intercompartmental balance (*B*).

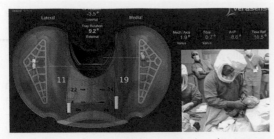

Fig. 9. The surgeon applies a posterior drawer test and sees minimal translation of the femoral contact points, indicating flexion gap stability.

stable knee, the contact points should remain in the central third of the bearing surface with minimal translation (**Fig. 9**).

Sagittal plane imbalance, which commonly leads to early revision, presents as excessive PCL tension or flexion gap instability.[32] Both intraoperative presentations are discernable, and can be corrected for, using sensor-embedded technology.

Excessive tension in the PCL is displayed through the sensor system as (1) an extreme posterior position of the femoral contact points, and (2) excessive loading in the posterior compartment during flexion. On application of a posterior drawer test, no excursion of the femorotibial contact points is detected.

If excessive loading presents in the posteriormedial compartment alone, this is indicative of required release of the PCL (**Fig. 10**).

When excessive loads are exhibited in both compartments simultaneously (symmetric imbalance), additional tibial slope can be added (**Fig. 11**).

Symmetric flexion instability can present in either the early or late postoperative phase, secondary to a rupture of the PCL.

Using the femoral contact-point tracking option of the sensor system, relative motion of the distal femur to the proximal tibia can be dynamically displayed during the posterior drawer test. Excessive excursion of the femoral contact points across the bearing surface (**Fig. 12**) and femoral contact points translating through the anterior third of the tibial trial are an indication of laxity in the PCL. Surgical correction requires the use of a thicker tibial insert, anterior-constrained insert, or a posteriorstabilized knee design.

Using sensor technology to guide the surgeon through appropriate sagittal plane correction, the subtleties in imbalance or suboptimal bone cuts can be accounted for, which otherwise may be overlooked by traditional methods of subjective surgeon "feel."

Malalignment

Malalignment leads to early failure and implant loosening,[33] and recent data have challenged the importance of the 3° range of alignment.[34] The outcomes presented in these studies may have been avoided with the ability to evaluate the critical elements of soft tissue balance and rotation,

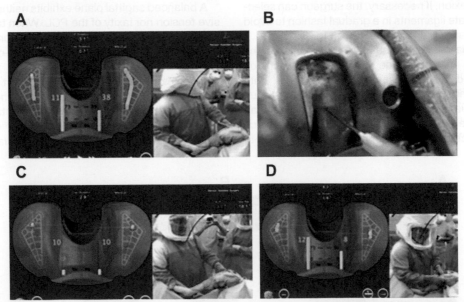

Fig. 10. (*A*) In this clinical case, excessive medial femoral rollback is seen with increased loads. (*B*) The PCL is dynamically pie-crusted and the knee re-cycled. (*C, D*) The flexion gap is now balanced, the medial femoral contact point centralized and a stable posterior drawer is seen to be stable on testing.

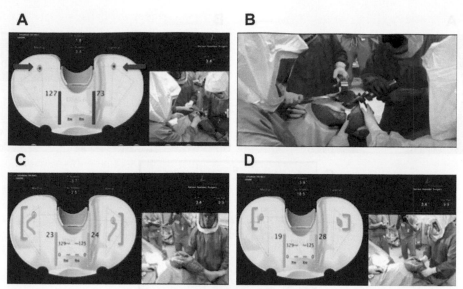

Fig. 11. (*A*) In this clinical case, excessive flexion loads are seen with excessive femoral rollback. The *arrows* are pointing out the location of femoral contact points on the tibial trial surface. (*B*) Two degrees of slope were added to optimize the flexion gap. (*C*) Rollback is optimized. (*D*) Posterior drawer shows excellent stability.

suboptimal data of which may be an indication of component malalignment (**Fig. 13**).

The advancement of implant design, polyethylene composite, and cementing techniques will affect implant function and longevity, although this will primarily depend on patient selection and surgical technique. Achieving a successful outcome is a complex amalgam of coronal and sagittal alignment, balance through a full range of motion, and optimized implant congruency and rotation.

THE FUTURE OF SOFT TISSUE BALANCING

The future of joint balancing will incorporate component rotation and alignment into the evaluation of soft tissue balance. Using one device that is constructed based on the geometric design of the implant will allow the surgeon to make real-time adjustments to all of these parameters, and witness how they affect patient soft tissue balance.

The ability to incorporate predictive shims will allow surgeons to evaluate, on a degree-by-degree scale, how varus-valgus alignment or tibial slope can alter the kinetic signature of the knee before they make adjustments. This assessment will lead to predictive modeling for each pathologic knee condition. The development of these algorithms will then enable the computer to help the surgeon decide which possible corrective maneuvers are most appropriate for current imbalance, while providing dynamic feedback as the corrective techniques are performed.

The large-scale collection of intraoperative data, coupled with patient demographic and surgical information, will help establish a national orthopedic registry. With a registry in place, a thorough analysis of outcomes, based on the multifactorial

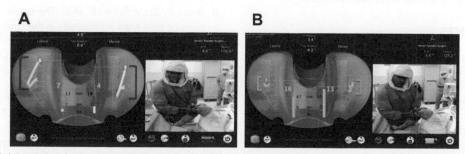

Fig. 12. (*A*) Excessive femoral translation is seen with a posterior drawer. (*B*) The surgeon adds 2 mm of thickness to the tibial trial and a stable flexion gap is achieved.

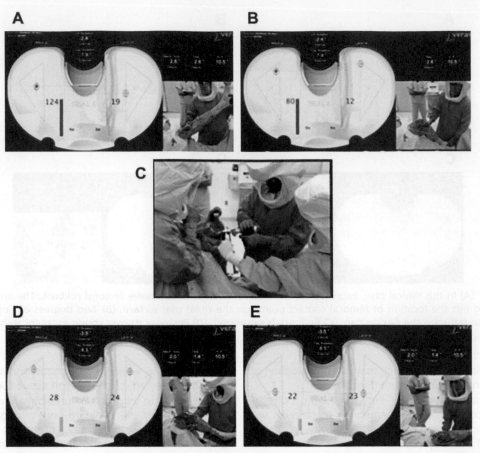

Fig. 13. (*A, B*) In this clinical case of tibia vara, the surgeon sees excessive loads medially in both the flexion and extension gaps. (*C*) Before performing any releases, he checks his tibial and femoral cuts and sees that he is in slight valgus, which adds to the medial tightness. He elects to add more varus to his tibial cut. (*D, E*) Optimal loads and gap kinematics have been achieved through a full range of motion.

aspects of knee replacement surgery, can be performed.

The full potential of sensor use in arthroplasty will be actualized when the implants themselves become embedded with microelectronics. This technique will help close the loop on how surgical technique directly affects the function and longevity of the total knee replacement.

REFERENCES

1. Berger R, Rosenberg A, Barden R, et al. Long-term followup of the Miller-Galante total knee replacement. Clin Orthop Relat Res 2001;388:58–67.

2. Keating E, Meding J, Faris P, et al. Long-term followup of nonmodular total knee replacements. Clin Orthop Relat Res 2002;404:34–9.

3. Sextro G, Berry D, Rand J. Total knee arthroplasty using cruciate-retaining kinematic condylar prosthesis. Clin Orthop Relat Res 2001;388:33–40.

4. Kurtz S, Ong K, Lau E, et al. Projections of primary and revision hip and knee arthroplasty in the united states from 2005 to 2030. J Bone Joint Surg Am 2007;89(4):780–5.

5. Bhandari M, Smith J, Miller L, et al. Clinical and economic burden of revision knee arthroplasty. Clin Med Insights Arthritis Musculoskelet Disord 2012;5: 89–94.

6. Bozic K, Kurtz S, Lau E, et al. The epidemiology of revision total knee arthroplasty in the United States. Clin Orthop Relat Res 2010;468:45–51.

7. Sharkey P, Hozack W, Rothman R, et al. Why are total knee arthroplasties failing today? Clin Orthop Relat Res 2002;404:7–13.

8. Fehring T, Odum S, Griffin W, et al. Early failures in total knee arthroplasty. Clin Orthop Relat Res 2001; 392:315–8.

9. Lonner J, Silliski J, Scott R. Prodromes of failure in total knee arthroplasty. J Arthroplasty 1999;14(4): 488–92.

10. Kuster M, Stachowiak G. Factors affecting polyethylene wear in total knee arthroplasty. Orthopedics 2002;25:235–42.

11. Lee S, Seong S, Lee S, et al. Outcomes of different types of total knee arthroplasty with identical femoral geometry. Knee Surg Relat Res 2012;24(4):214–20.

12. Gallo J, Goodman S, Konttinen Y, et al. Osteolysis around total knee arthroplasty: a review of pathogenic mechanisms. Acta Biomater 2013;9(9):8046–58.

13. Barrack R, Schrader T, Bertot A. Component rotation and anterior knee pain after total knee arthroplasty. Clin Orthop Relat Res 2001;392:46–55.

14. Berger R, Crossett L, Jacobs J, et al. Malrotation causing patellofemoral complications after total knee arthroplasty. Clin Orthop Relat Res 1998;356:144–53.

15. Dennis D, Komistek R, Kim R. Gap balancing versus measured resection technique for total knee arthroplasty. Clin Orthop Relat Res 2010;468:102–7.

16. Heesterbeek P, Keijsers N, Jacobs W, et al. Posterior cruciate ligament recruitment affects anteroposterior translation during flexion gap distraction in total knee replacement. Acta Orthop 2010;81(4):471–7.

17. Mihalko W, Whiteside L, Krackow K. Comparison of ligament-balancing techniques during total knee arthroplasty. J Bone Joint Surg Am 2003;85:132–5.

18. Scuderi G, Komistek R, Dennis D, et al. The impact of femoral component malrotation in total knee arthroplasty. Clin Orthop Relat Res 2003;410:148–54.

19. Whiteside L, Arima J. The anteroposterior axis for femoral rotational alignment in valgus total knee arthroplasty. Clin Orthop Relat Res 1995;321:168–72.

20. Bellemans J, Vandenneucker H, Van Lauwe J, et al. New surgical technique for medial collateral ligament balancing. J Arthroplasty 2010;25(7):1151–6.

21. Boldt J, Stiehl J, Hodler J, et al. Femoral component rotation and arthrofibrosis following mobile-bearing total knee arthroplasty. Int Orthop 2006;30:420–5.

22. Crossett L. Fixed versus mobile-bearing total knee arthroplasty: technical issues and surgical tips. Orthopedics 2002;25:251–6.

23. Incavo S, Wild J, Coughlin K, et al. Early revision for component malrotation in total knee arthroplasty. Clin Orthop Relat Res 2007;13:455–72.

24. Lutzner J, Krummenauer F, Gunther KP, et al. Rotational alignment of the tibial component in total knee arthroplasty is better at the medial third f the tibial tuberosity than at the medial border. BMC Musculoskelet Disord 2010;11(57):1–7.

25. Howell S, Hodapp E, Vernace J, et al. Are undesirable contact kinematics minimized after kinematically aligned total knee arthroplasty? An intersurgeon analysis of consecutive patients. Knee Surg Sports Traumatol Arthrosc 2012;21(10):2281–7.

26. Hutter E, Granger J, Beal M. Is there a gold standard for TKA tibial component rotational alignment? Clin Orthop Relat Res 2013;471(5):1646–53.

27. Rossi R, Bruzzone M, Bonasia D, et al. Evaluation of tibial rotational alignment in total knee arthroplasty: a cadaver study. Knee Surg Sports Traumatol Arthrosc 2002;18:889–93.

28. Sun T, Lu H, Hong N, et al. Bony landmarks and rotational alignment in total knee arthroplasty for Chinese osteoarthritic knees with varus and valgus deformities. J Arthroplasty 2009;24:427–31.

29. Uehara K, Kadoya Y, Kobayashi A, et al. Bone anatomy and rotational alignment in total knee arthroplasty. Clin Orthop Relat Res 2002;402:196–201.

30. Golladay G, Roche M, Elson L, et al. Variability of tibial tray rotation: how accurate are our most reliable methods? Presented at the annual meeting of the International Congress for Joint Replacement West. Napa Valley, June 6, 2013.

31. Jerry G, Dounchis J, Golladay G. Computer-assisted orthopaedic surgery during TKA is insufficient for ensuring ideal joint reconstruction. Presented at the annual meeting of the International Congress for Joint Replacement West. Napa Valley, June 6, 2013.

32. Scott R, Chmell M. Balancing the posterior cruciate ligament during cruciate-retaining fixed and mobile-bearing total knee arthroplasty. J Arthroplasty 2008;23(4):605–8.

33. Dossett H, Swartz G, Estrada N, et al. Kinematically versus mechanically aligned total knee arthroplasty. Orthopedics 2012;35(2):160–9.

34. Parratte S, Pagnano M, Trousdale R, et al. Effect of post-operative mechanical axis alignment on the fifteen-year survival of modern, cemented total knee replacements. J Bone Joint Surg Am 2010;92(12):2143–9.

Total Knee Arthroplasty with a Novel Navigation System Within the Surgical Field

Giles R. Scuderi, MD[a],*, Michel Fallaha, MD[b], Vincent Masse, MD[b], Patrick Lavigne, MD, PhD[b], Louis-Philippe Amiot, MD, MSc[c], Marie-Josee Berthiaume, MD[b]

KEYWORDS

- Total knee arthroplasty • Computer navigation • Total knee alignment • Smart instrumentation

KEY POINTS

- A new novel navigation system used within the surgical field has demonstrated reproducible accuracy in component alignment.
- All orientation information is captured by small electronic pods and transmitted via a local wireless (Wi-Fi) network, which directs the surgical workflow automatically to the femoral and tibial resection instruments.
- The system demonstrates accuracy comparable to optical navigation.
- iAssist provides a novel navigation system for all users. For surgeons who prefer conventional instrumentation, the electronic pods provide intelligence and accuracy to the resection guide, whereas for surgeons who prefer computer navigation, this system provides the same accuracy with simplicity.

INTRODUCTION

Over the past years, the effect of alignment on implant survival has been well documented,[1–4] with its influence on implant survival, component loosening, and clinical outcome scores. Numerous publications have documented the accuracy of computer-assisted navigation with knee arthroplasty,[5–8] with some early postoperative benefits in recuperation, clinical function,[9,10] and blood loss.[11]

Total knee arthroplasty navigation systems have been around since 1995 and have taken various forms: image-based navigation, imageless navigation, fluoroscopy-based navigation, electromagnetic navigation, and optical navigation. Adoption of these systems in the overall number of procedures is still limited to approximately 5%, mostly because of the perceived complexity and the additional time required in the use of these systems.

Patient-specific instruments (PSI) appeared around 2006 and have reached a greater use rate than computer navigation.[12–15] The surgical workflow with PSI is simpler than navigation, but requires preoperative imaging—either magnetic resonance imaging (MRI) or computed tomography (CT)—presurgical planning, and manufacturing of the resection guides. These personalized instruments are attractive, but have intraoperative obstacles that are not infrequently encountered, and therefore deviations from the preoperative plan may be necessary. In addition, once the bone is resected, there is no ability to validate the bone cuts.

GRS, MF and VM are the consultants for Zimmer Orthopedics, L-PA is an employee for Zimmer Orthopedics.
[a] Insall Scott Kelly Institute, 210 East 64th Street, New York, NY 10065, USA; [b] Orthopedic Department, Hopital Maisonneuve-Rosemont, 5415 Boul de l'Assomption, Montreal, H1T 2M4, Canada; [c] Zimmer CAS, 75 Queen Street, Montreal, H3C 2N6, Canada
* Corresponding author.
E-mail address: grscuderi@aol.com

More recently, navigation systems have been developed using inertial electronic components,[16–18] which simplifies the tracking process, especially when compared with optical navigation systems. One of these new navigation systems is iAssist (Zimmer, Inc., Warsaw, IN, USA), which is an alignment system designed with the user interface built into disposable electronic pods that attach onto the femoral and tibial resection instruments. Within these pods are inertial electronic components or gyroscopes that exchange information using a secure local wireless (Wi-Fi) channel. After capture of the necessary data during the procedure, the alignment information is displayed to the surgeon directly on the pods within the surgical field. These pods are attached to either the femoral or tibial resection guides, which then guide the resection at the appropriate angles in both the coronal and sagittal planes. After bone resection, the accuracy of the alignment can be validated, confirming the position of both the femoral and tibial components.

The surgical workflow follows the classic method of femoral and tibia bone resection with each bone resected independently along the mechanical axis. The following section describes the surgical technique for the iAssist system.

Tibial Coordinate System Registration

As with other navigation systems, the coordinate system for each bone must be defined. For the iAssist system, an extramedullary tibial guide with an electronic digitizing pod secured to the tibia will identify the mechanical axis and guide the bone resection. The proximal position of the guide is positioned between the tibial spines in the center of the tibial joint surface. Two spikes secure the guide in this region. The distal portion of the alignment guide is mounted with a self-centering claw, which is positioned on the malleoli and fixes the instrument at the center of the ankle joint. The digitizer is then oriented in line with the medial third of the tibial tuberosity and fixed rigidly in place. Once secure, the alignment guide is positioned along the mechanical axis, as seen in **Fig. 1**A. The angular relationship between the electronic pod of the digitizer and the bone reference is registered by the system through 3 movements of the limb: abduction, adduction, and neutral position. This function activates the inertial mechanism and creates the coordinate system required for navigation. Once the information has been registered, the digitizer is removed and the data are transferred wirelessly to the electronic pod on the tibial cutting guide, which has 2 knobs to adjust the varus/valgus alignment and the tibial slope. The electronic pod, viewed entirely within the operative field, accurately reports the data with incremental visual cues, including red lights when out of alignment and green lights when the cutting guide is within the desired alignment and slope (see **Fig. 1**B). Once the position of the resection guide is satisfactory, the depth of resection is

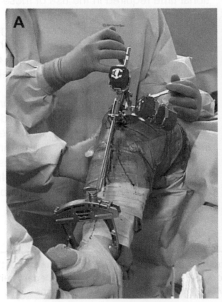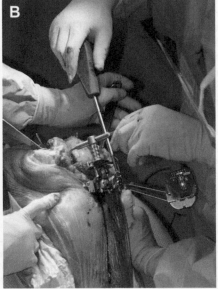

Fig. 1. (*A*) The tibia digitizer has been impacted to the proximal articular surface and fixed to the malleoli with its self-centering claw. On the medial side, a bone reference pod has been fixed just below the articular line. (*B*) Intraoperative view of the surgeon adjusting a tibial cut guide. A green light is clearly visible on the iAssist device, indicating proper varus/valgus orientation and slope.

manually set and the cutting guide is secured to the proximal tibia, which is then cut in the usual fashion. After resection, the alignment and slope of the proximal tibial surface can be validated with an electronic pod. If any adjustment to the resection is needed, it can be performed at this time and the accuracy of the resection rechecked with the electronic validation tool.

Femoral Coordinate System Registration

Similar to most optical navigation systems, the mechanical axis is determined by the anatomically located center of the distal femur and the kinematic determination of the femoral hip center. A line connecting those 2 landmarks then defines the mechanical axis of the femur.

With the iAssist system, a bone spike is impacted into the distal femoral sulcus approximately 10 mm anterior to the posterior cruciate ligament, in the anatomic location of the distal femoral mechanical axis. A sleeve with an electronic pod attached is then inserted over the spike and fixed to the trochlear groove. The femoral hip center is then registered through multiple stop-and-go movements by the surgeon. The system provides an auditory cue when the bone is stopped, signaling the surgeon to proceed to the next movement. Multiple acquisitions are taken and recorded by the electronic pod, and the mechanical axis of the femur is acquired. The distal femoral resection guide with a separate electronic pod is then coupled to the femoral spike. The alignment information from the first pod is transferred wirelessly to the second pod, which guides the resection of the distal femur, including the mechanical axis and flexion. The electronic pod, viewed entirely within the operative field, accurately reports the data with incremental visual cues, including red lights when out of alignment and green lights when the cutting guide is within the desired alignment and flexion (**Fig. 2**). Once the position of the resection guide is satisfactory, the depth of resection is set and the cutting guide is secured to the distal femur. The femoral spike is then removed and the distal femur is resected in the usual fashion. After resection, the alignment and flexion of the distal femur surface can be validated with an electronic pod. If any adjustments to the resection are needed, these can be performed at this time and the accuracy of the resection rechecked with the electronic validation tool.

Preclinical Validation Study

Preclinical validation was performed with a comparative study on cadaveric specimens using an optical navigation system and iAssist

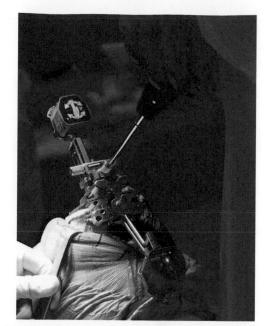

Fig. 2. View of the femur during adjustment: the bone reference (*top blue pod*) provides the anchor point for the adjustment mechanism. The surgeon adjusts the cut guide until both lights of the lower pod turn green.

simultaneously. The intent was to compare the values for both the femoral and tibial resections. In addition, the limb alignment was assessed with fluoroscopic images of the whole limb. The mechanical axes were compared on a bone-to-bone basis.

For all optical measurements, a Navitrack (Zimmer, Inc.) system running TKR 3.2 was used. As required with the optical navigation protocol, bone trackers were installed on both the femur and the tibia, and bone registrations performed. The iAssist system was then used as described earlier concurrently with the optical system. The iAssist cut guide was adjusted to position the resection guides in a neutral mechanical axis for both the femur and the tibia. The preselected tibial slope was adjusted to 7° and the femoral flexion angle was preselected to 3°. Before any bone cuts were made, the optical navigation system was used to register the orientation of the cut guide and any discrepancy was noted. After bone cuts were made, iAssist was used to measure and validate the resected bone surfaces, and the optical navigation system was used to measure the same final bone surface; any discrepancies with the iAssist system were noted.

After the validated bone resection, each cadaver knee had a posterior stabilized total knee arthroplasty implanted. Each knee then underwent

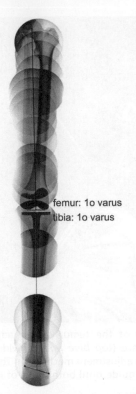

femur: 1o varus
tibia: 1o varus

Fig. 3. Fluoroscopy stitching of multiple images to produce a long-leg femur and tibia radiograph. In this example, both femoral and tibial components are placed with 1° of varus.

fluoroscopic measurements with an OEC 9600 C-Arm (General Electric, Fairfield, CT, USA). Multiple fluoroscopic images were taken from the ankle to the head of the femur. Specific software was used to stitch the images together to obtain the equivalent of a long-leg radiograph (**Fig. 3**). Mechanical axes were computed for the femur and then for the tibia. Discrepancies were recorded and compared with the angles obtained with the optical navigation system.

Preclinical results obtained from 8 cadaveric specimens are documented on **Table 1**. Comparison of optical navigation and iAssist measurements showed an average error of 0.5°. Similar accuracies were obtained with fluoroscopic

measurements, but standard deviations tended to be smaller with this group.

Early Clinical Validation Study

After approval from the ethics committee, a prospective randomized study using iAssist navigation was initiated. A total of 25 patients were enrolled in each arm of the study and the results from the first 14 are being reported. After implantation of the total knee arthroplasty, the accuracy of the bone cuts was evaluated using a supine postoperative CT scan of the entire lower limb. To measure bone cuts as accurately as possible, a series of landmarks were taken on multiaxial views of the femur and the tibia, as used previously in the Perth protocol.[19] The landmark voxel coordinates were then used to compute the coordinate system of the femur and tibia, and the position of the implants relative to their respective bone. The difference between values shown intraoperatively during bone cut validation and the bone cuts measured on CT scans were computed. All data analysis was performed on Excel (Microsoft Corporation, Redmond, WA, USA).

The early clinical results in this study for the first 14 patients are shown in **Tables 2** and **3** demonstrating the intraoperative validation values for the femur and tibia, respectively, compared with the postoperative CT measurements. The average error on femoral validation values is −0.22° ± 0.83° for varus/valgus and 0.39° ± 0.95° for flexion/extension (see **Table 2**). The average error on tibial validation values is 0.74° ± 1.07° for varus/valgus and −0.05° ± 0.78° for slope (see **Table 3**).

DISCUSSION

The debate about the usability of computers in the surgical field is still ongoing. Most surgeons are receptive to the idea as long as it does not impede the workflow, improves their accuracy, and is ergonomically acceptable. Optical navigation has advanced in the past 15 years in terms of usability, but the fundamental problems remain: capital expense, multiple landmarking, placement of additional pins for the trackers, and line-of-sight

Table 1
Preclinical results: accuracy of iAssist compared with optical navigation and fluoroscopy

	Tibia Varus/Valgus	Tibia Slope	Femur Varus/Valgus	Femur Flexion/Extension
Discrepancy between optical navigation and iAssist	0.5 ± 1.4° (n = 8)	0.5 ± 0.9° (n = 8)	0.0 ± 0.5° (n = 8)	0.1 ± 0.7° (n = 8)
Discrepancy between fluoroscopy and iAssist	0.2 ± 1.3° (n = 8)		0.5 ± 0.7° (n = 8)	

Table 2
Accuracy of femur measurements

Patient	Varus (+) Valgus (–)			Flexion (+) Extension (–)		
	iAssist	CT	Error	iAssist	CT	Error
1	−0.8	−1.20	−0.40	2.8	4.50	1.70
2	0.3	0.70	0.40	−0.1	1.20	1.30
3	−0.2	−0.90	−0.70	1.4	2.00	0.60
4	−0.4	−0.70	−0.30	4.4	4.60	0.20
5	−0.5	0.20	0.69	3.0	2.00	−1.00
6	−0.5	−1.30	−0.80	2.9	4.00	1.10
7	0.4	1.30	0.90	7.5	7.70	0.20
8	0.0	0.40	0.40	3.7	2.40	−1.30
9	0.2	0.70	0.50	1.6	2.00	0.40
10	0.4	1.30	0.90	0.7	1.40	0.70
11	0.3	−1.10	−1.41	0.8	1.50	0.74
12	1.5	0.20	−1.34	0.1	0.70	0.61
13	0.7	0.00	−0.68	3.2	4.40	1.24
14	0.3	−0.90	−1.17	1.6	1.10	−0.53
		Average: −0.22 SD: 0.83			Average: 0.39 SD: 0.95	

issues with the tracking system. These issues are negated with iAssist because of the ease of use with essentially smart conventional instrumentation. Having the navigation system completely within the operative field facilitates the workflow and is a real benefit for the surgeon. The electronic pods mounted on the surgical instruments direct the workflow with reproducible accuracy. Small magnets on key instrument surfaces detect the assembly and disassembly of neighboring

Table 3
Accuracy of tibia measurements

Patient	Varus (+) Valgus (–)			Slope		
	iAssist	CT	Error	iAssist	CT	Error
1	−0.4	−0.20	0.20	4.8	4.30	−0.50
2	0.9	0.60	−0.30	5.3	4.60	−0.70
3	−0.7	−1.20	−0.50	6.3	5.70	−0.60
4	−0.6	0.10	0.70	3.6	4.30	0.70
5	−0.4	−0.50	−0.10	7.0	6.20	−0.80
6	−0.1	2.30	2.40	4.9	5.30	0.40
7	0.6	1.30	0.70	7.3	6.70	−0.60
8	1.6	2.30	0.70	7.0	8.20	1.20
9	−2.4	0.50	2.90	6.6	7.20	0.60
10	0.2	0.50	0.30	6.4	5.70	−0.70
11	−0.3	0.10	0.39	5.7	5.40	−0.32
12	−1.6	0.80	2.38	9.6	9.80	0.18
13	0.3	0.20	−0.12	6.8	8.20	1.37
14	0.0	0.80	0.77	6.3	5.40	−0.93
		Average: 0.74 SD: 1.07			Average: −0.05 SD: 0.78	

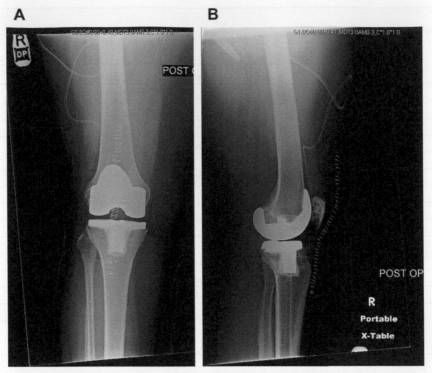

Fig. 4. Anteroposterior (*A*) and lateral (*B*) radiograph of total knee arthroplasty performed with iAssist.

instruments and direct the software through the appropriate surgical steps. Although each electronic pod functions similar to an intraoperative monitor, a computer controller is also present in the operating room and is monitored by the surgical support staff.

Reproducible accuracy with iAssist was obtained in the preclinical validation phase. Discrepancies between iAssist and optical navigation were always small (<0.5°). Fluoroscopic validation also provided the same level of accuracy. This finding underlines the correspondence between the different methods used to build coordinate systems and the ultimate check with reality.

Initial clinical values measured on CT showed a good correlation to actual validation measurements from the iAssist system. The femoral mechanical axis showed an average accuracy of 0.4°± 0.95° between the validated bone surface and the postoperative CT. Tibial measurements of the mechanical axis also proved accurate, with an average error of 0.70° ± 1.07°. Tibial slope results were reproducible, with errors of −0.05° ± 0.78°. Current clinical and radiographic analysis has demonstrated reproducible accuracy in component alignment (**Fig. 4**).

iAssist provides a novel navigation system for all users. For surgeons who prefer conventional instrumentation, the electronic pods provide

intelligence and accuracy to the resection guide, whereas for surgeons who prefer computer navigation, this system provides the same accuracy with simplicity.

REFERENCES

1. Ritter MA, Davis KE, Meding JB, et al. The effect of alignment and BMI on failure of total knee replacement. J Bone Joint Surg Am 2011;93(17):1588–96.
2. Sikorski JM. Alignment in total knee replacement. J Bone Joint Surg Br 2008;90(9):1121–7.
3. Ritter MA. The Anatomical Graduated Component total knee replacement: a long-term evaluation with 20-year survival analysis. J Bone Joint Surg Br 2009;91(6):745–9.
4. Petersen TL, Engh GA. Radiographic assessment of knee alignment after total knee arthroplasty. J Arthroplasty 1988;3(1):67–72.
5. Weng YJ, Hsu RW, Hsu WH, et al. Comparison of computer-assisted navigation and conventional instrumentation for bilateral total knee arthroplasty. J Arthroplasty 2009;24(5):668–73.
6. Mullaji A, Shetty GM. Computer-assisted total knee arthroplasty for arthritis with extra-articular deformity. J Arthroplasty 2009;24(8):1164–9.e1.
7. Biasca N, Schneider TO, Bungartz M, et al. Minimally invasive computer-navigated total knee arthroplasty. Orthop Clin North Am 2009;40(4):537–63.

8. Carter RE 3rd, Rush PF, Smid JA, et al. Experience with computer-assisted navigation for total knee arthroplasty in a community setting. J Arthroplasty 2008;23(5):707–13.

9. Dutton AQ, Yeo SJ. Computer-assisted minimally invasive total knee arthroplasty compared with standard total knee arthroplasty. Surgical technique. J Bone Joint Surg Am 2009;91(Suppl 2 Pt 1):116–30.

10. Choong PF, Dowsey MM, Stoney JD, et al. Does accurate anatomical alignment result in better function and quality of life? Comparing conventional and computer-assisted total knee arthroplasty. J Arthroplasty 2009;24(4):560–9.

11. Conteduca F, Massai F, Iorio R, et al. Blood loss in computer-assisted mobile bearing total knee arthroplasty. A comparison of computer-assisted surgery with a conventional technique. Int Orthop 2009; 33(6):1609–13.

12. Daniilidis K, Tibesku CO. A comparison of conventional and patient-specific instruments in total knee arthroplasty. Int Orthop 2013. [Epub ahead of print].

13. Daniilidis K, Tibesku CO. Frontal plane alignment after total knee arthroplasty using patient-specific instruments. Int Orthop 2013;37(1):45–50.

14. Hendel MD, Bryan JA, Barsoum WK, et al. Comparison of patient-specific instruments with standard surgical instruments in determining glenoid component position: a randomized prospective clinical trial. J Bone Joint Surg Am 2012;94(23):2167–75.

15. Stevens A, Beurskens A, Köke A, et al. The use of patient-specific measurement instruments in the process of goal-setting: a systematic review of available instruments and their feasibility. Clin Rehabil 2013;27(11):1005–19.

16. Nam D, Weeks KD, Reinhardt KR, et al. Accelerometer-based, portable navigation vs imageless, large-console computer-assisted navigation in total knee arthroplasty: a comparison of radiographic results. J Arthroplasty 2013;28(2):255–61.

17. Nam D, Jerabek SA, Haughom B, et al. Radiographic analysis of a hand-held surgical navigation system for tibial resection in total knee arthroplasty. J Arthroplasty 2011;26(8):1527–33.

18. Khan H, Walker PS, Zuckerman JD, et al. The potential of accelerometers in the evaluation of stability of total knee arthroplasty. J Arthroplasty 2013;28(3): 459–62.

19. Chauhan SK, Clark GW, Lloyd S, et al. Computer-assisted total knee replacement. A controlled cadaver study using a multi-parameter quantitative CT assessment of alignment (the Perth CT Protocol). J Bone Joint Surg Br 2004;86(6):818–23.

Soft Tissue Balance in Total Knee Arthroplasty with a Force Sensor

David A. Camarata, MD

KEYWORDS

- eLibra Dynamic Ligament Balancing Device • Medial collateral ligament • Lateral collateral ligament
- Transepicondylar axis • Whiteside line • Femoral component • External rotation

KEY POINTS

- The eLibra device uses quantitative real-time data to balance the knee as opposed to static landmarks for external rotation of the femoral component.
- The medial collateral ligament (MCL) and lateral collateral ligament (LCL) are balanced through bone cuts rather than ligament releases.
- The device is simple to use, highly accurate, and reproducible.
- Use of this device greatly reduces the need for ligament releases and confirms precise balance when used in combination with computer-assisted navigation, patient-specific cutting guides, or conventional arthroplasty.

INTRODUCTION

Total knee arthroplasty (TKA) remains one of the most successful surgical procedures in the world. It is a clinical fact that this procedure, properly performed, improves pain, increases range of motion, and improves the quality of life for patients undergoing this procedure. The success of TKA largely depends on restoration of the integrity of the articular surfaces of the knee joint as well as realignment of the entire lower extremity to a neutral or an anatomic mechanical axis.[1–4]

The 2 critical elements of TKA, in terms of restoration of the joint surfaces and realignment of the limb, are the bone cuts and appropriate and reproducible soft tissue balancing, particularly in flexion. Initially, the procedure relied on rudimentary instruments to achieve appropriate osteotomies. Over the past 2 to 3 decades, there have been major advances in the instruments available to perform correct and reproducible bony cuts.

Initially, intramedullary instrumentation was shown particularly accurate in terms of bony resurfacing. This led to the development of extramedullary guides to do the same.

Over the past 10 years, there have been enormous advances in bone preparation with the development of computer-assisted navigation and validation techniques as well as, recently, the advent of image-guided preoperative patient-specific instrumentation systems. These systems use preoperative MRI- or CT-based technology to rapidly produce a set of cutting jigs specifically designed to reproduce a patient's normal knee anatomy, eliminating the need for intramedullary or extramedullary preparation and shown to be highly accurate and to reduce outliers.[5,6]

Despite these advances in bone preparation, little has been done to assist surgeons in appropriate soft tissue balancing. Precise osteotomies ensure appropriate prosthetic fit but do little to

D.A. Camarata is a paid consultant by Zimmer Inc and serves as an Instructor in the Zimmer Institute for Knee technologies and revision knee replacement.
Ortho Arizona: Arizona Bone and Joint Specialists, 5620 East Bell Road, Scottsdale, AZ 85254, USA
E-mail address: davecamarata@cox.net

Orthop Clin N Am 45 (2014) 175–184
http://dx.doi.org/10.1016/j.ocl.2013.12.001

ensure ligamentous stability and balance. Instability and improper balance have been shown to lead to condylar liftoff, flexion instability, accelerated prosthetic wear, aseptic loosening, patellar maltracking, anterior knee pain, and overall increase in mechanical failure.[7–10]

Soft tissue balance remains largely technique driven and highly dependent on the discretion of the operative surgeon. Osteotomies are usually completed; then, the surgeon ensures appropriate range of motion and stability by individually testing the MCL, LCL, and anterior-to-posterior stability in extension, flexion, and throughout the range of motion. Balance is then achieved through ligamentous releases and/or repeat osteotomies. Typically, after years of experience and numerous procedures, a surgeon develops the ability to accurately assess stability in the varus/valgus and anterior/posterior planes.

This article discusses a new intraoperative device designed to assist surgeons with soft tissue balance primarily in flexion. The eLibra Dynamic Knee Balancing System (Zimmer, Warsaw, Indiana) provides a quantitative way to measure the compressive forces across the knee joint in the medial and lateral compartments in flexion and extension. The surgeon then reverses the traditional order of steps in the surgery, balancing the flexion space with the aid of the eLibra to externally rotate the trial component before the finishing femoral anteroposterior (AP) cuts are made. Rather than relying on the typical bone landmarks of 3° of posterior condylar rotation, Whiteside line, or the transepicondylar axis (TEA), flexion balanced is achieved by rotating the femoral trial to equalize compressive forces relative to the resected tibia on the force sensor.

This process takes into account 3 critical anatomic structures: the tibial osteotomy in terms of varus valgus alignment, the MCL, and the LCL. All have been shown of primary importance in soft tissue balancing.

After equalization of the compressive forces on both sides of the joint in 90° of flexion, the final femoral cuts are completed prior to any releases, eliminating or minimizing the need for soft tissue balancing after implantation of the trial or actual components. Dynamic balance is then achieved through a process termed, *balanced resection*, which is a combination of gap balancing and measured resection techniques.

This article describes the eLibra device and its application in terms of a quantitative measure of gap balancing. This device gives real-time objective data, similar to navigation data, with reference to the medial and lateral compressive forces across the joint.

In describing the device, 4 learning objectives are focused on:

1. Description of the normal balancing forces across the knee joint in TKA, including traditional means of achieving balance
2. Description of the design rationale and technical specifications of the eLibra Dynamic Knee Balancing System
3. The use of the eLibra Dynamic Knee Balancing Knee System to balance the knee and obtain objective data regarding medial and lateral compressive forces across the knee joint in flexion and extension
4. Early results using this device in the published literature

KNEE JOINT STABILITY AND ACHIEVING BALANCE

The knee joint is an inherently unstable articulation and relies on both static and dynamic stabilizers to achieve stability. Static stabilizers are the MCL, the LCL, the anterior and posterior cruciate ligaments, and the posterior capsule. Current total knee designs sacrifice the anterior and/or the posterior cruciate ligaments, relying on inherent prosthetic stability for anterior-to-posterior constraint with a dished tibial articular polyethylene or a post-and-cam mechanism. The medial lateral stability comprises the MCL and LCL and to some extent the posterior capsule in extension. Appropriate balance of these structures is critical to overall stability of the prosthetic joint, and imbalance of these structures can lead to instability, particularly in flexion; accelerated wear; and overall poor performance of the arthroplasty.[11] Both the MCL and the LCL can be divided into anterior and posterior halves: the anterior half is maximally tight inflexion and the posterior half is tight in full extension. Many investigators have postulated that arthritis and joint destruction is a disease of not only the condylar surfaces but also the ligaments themselves.[12] Thus TKA must address the ligaments as well. In the extreme, this process involves complete stripping of the entire posterior medial corner or the lateral structures in a tight valgus knee. The author believes that the amount of ligamentous release can be and should be dictated by the preexisting varus or valgus deformity and the ability to passively correct the deformity preoperatively. A passively correctible deformity requires little or no ligamentous releases and can usually be completely balanced through the bone cuts with the eLibra. A fixed varus or valgus deformity most likely requires some release to correct the deformity and balance the flexion and extension gaps.

There are also several dynamic stabilizers of the knee joint. The anterior structures include the quadriceps muscle and tendon, the patella, and the patellar ligament, collectively known as the extensor mechanism. The posterior structures include the medial and lateral hamstrings, which actively flex the joint, resist in extension, and provide some dynamic rotational stability. Also, the popliteus muscle assists in controlling internal rotation of the femur on the tibia.

It is the complex interplay between the static and dynamic stabilizers of the knee joint that is critical to the medial and lateral balance of the prosthetic knee joint. The interplay is so complex that individually measuring each component is impossible. This interplay is where the eLibra helps surgeons. Balance is achieved through bone cuts, not violation of the soft tissue. The balance is ensured prior to the osteotomies and confirmed with precise objective feedback.

TRADITIONAL BALANCING TECHNIQUES

Soft tissue balance in knee arthroplasty has 2 schools of thought: measured resection versus gap balancing. Both methods are designed to create a symmetric flexion space by resection of the posterior condyles to match the symmetric extension space created by the distal femoral osteotomy.

The measured resection technique relies on 1 or all of 3 anatomic bony references to achieve resection:

1. TEA
2. Posterior femoral condyles
3. Anterior posterior axis (Whiteside line)

Gap balancing relies on the femoral component positioned parallel to the resected proximal tibia with each collateral ligament equally tensioned in flexion. This typically requires the use of tensiometers or laminar spreaders and is inherently subjective, requires experience, and is difficult to master.

The eLibra device relies on ligament tensioning but in an objective clinically relevant manner (**Fig. 1**).

PITFALLS WITH MEASURED RESECTION TECHNIQUE
Transepicondylar Axis

The TEA is the axis positioned perpendicular to the tibial mechanical axis in 90° of flexion. For this reason, it is an excellent reference for femoral component rotation.[13] This theory has been supported by clinical research demonstrating a reduced incidence and reduced magnitude of femoral liftoff in deep flexion.[14] It is sometimes difficult, however, intraoperatively to adequately define the femoral epicondyles, particularly in

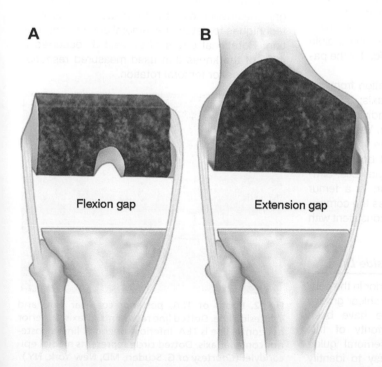

A Flexion gap

B Extension gap

Fig. 1. Flexion gap and extension gap. (*A*) Flexion gap composed of posterior femoral condyles and tibial surface. (*B*) Extension gap composed of distal femoral condyles and tibial surface. (*From* Kang N, Scuderi GR. Sizing and balancing: gap technique vs. measured resection. In: Brown TE, Cui Q, Mihalko WM, et al, editors. Arthritis and Arthroplasty: The Knee. 1st Edition. Philadelphia: Saunders; 2009; with permission.)

a limited incision arthroplasty, which can lead to flexion gap asymmetry.

Kinzell and colleagues[15] reported on a series of 74 knees, which involved marking the epicondyles intraoperatively with pins that were evaluated with postoperative CT scans for accuracy of epicondyle identification. Only 75% or the pins correctly identified the epicondyles to within 3°. There was also a wide range of error from 6° of external rotation to 11° of internal rotation.

Another study by Yau and colleagues[16] confirmed significant variability in surgeon ability to correctly identify the TEA, with an error range of 28°. Even if this axis is properly identified, it does not take into account any ligament tension, which can require releases to balance the space.

Posterior Femoral Condyles

A horizontal line connecting the most inferior point of the condyles to each other defines the posterior condylar axis. This line has been shown by several studies consistently 3° to 4° internally rotated to the TEA.[17] Many manufacturers of instrumentation systems have designed jigs to account for this axis by placing the femoral cutting guides into 3° or 4° of external rotation in reference to the posterior condylar axis.

This axis is a good approximation but has 2 major pitfalls.

1. The valgus knee typically has a hypoplastic lateral femoral condyle. Use of the posterior condylar axis in this situation leads to severe internal rotation of the femoral component, making true ligament balance almost impossible and creating suboptimal kinematics for the patella femoral joint.
2. In addition, there is a wide variation from the TEA to the posterior condylar axis; 3° or 4° are mean values and can miss individual rotational variability in certain femurs. Variability of rotation has been shown between 1° internally rotated to 10° externally rotated between the TEA and posterior femoral condylar axis. Simply using 3° of external rotation in a femur with a TEA of 10° internally rotates the component 7°. Again, this situation is inconsistent with a symmetric flexion gap.

The Anteroposterior Axis (Whiteside Line)

This axis runs from anterior to posterior in the center of the deepest portion of the trochlear groove to the intercondylar notch. There have been studies demonstrating the superiority of this method with placement of the femoral guide perpendicular to this line. It is easy to identify

and proponents of this method cite ease of balance and improved patellar tracking as its benefits.[18] There can be significant interobserver error in placement of the femoral component, however, and many studies reveal significant rotational malallignment when using this axis. Yau and colleagues[19] found a 32° range of error when using the AP axis (17° of internal rotation to 15° of external rotation.) An additional study by Nagamine and colleagues[20] revealed significant external rotation errors in varus knees with severe medial compartment arthrosis (**Fig. 2**).

GAP BALANCING TECHNIQUE

The gap balancing technique is defined as placing the femoral component parallel to the resected proximal tibia with both the MCL complex and the LCL complex, balanced equally with the use of tensiometers, laminar spreaders, or other tension devices. Advocates of gap balancing report better flexion stability, patellar tracking, and reproducibility of the technique for use in placement of the femoral component rotation.[7] This technique relies on pure ligament tension to place the femoral component parallel to the cut tibial surface prior to the femoral AP osteotomy, in contradistinction to the measured resection techniques, which rely only on anatomic static landmarks. These techniques essentially miss the entire process of ligamentous balancing by not addressing ligament tension until after the bone cuts are made.

Fehring,[21] in a study of 100 knees, compared gap balancing directly to measured resection techniques to determine femoral component rotation. Rotational errors of at least 3° occurred in 45% of the knees that used measured resection techniques for femoral rotation.

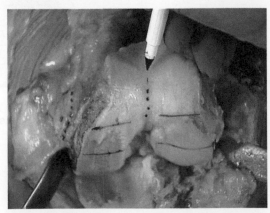

Fig. 2. Photo of TEA, posterior condylar axis, and Whiteside line. Dotted line represents AP axis. Superior horizontal line is TEA. Inferior horizontal line is posterior condylar axis. Dotted circle represents medial epicondyle. (*Courtesy of* G. Scuderi, MD, New York, NY.)

Dennis and colleagues[7] used computer-assisted navigational techniques to evaluate 212 patients undergoing TKA. The TEA, AP line, and posterior condylar axis were all registered and then compared with the gap balancing technique.

There was a wide variability in all 3 measured resection techniques to gap balancing. When using the TEA for rotation, the femoral component was positioned at a mean of 0.9° externally rotated to the gap balance technique (with a range of 12° internal to 16° externally rotated). The TEA method was within 3° of the gap balance method in only 43% of cases.

Using the AP axis had similar results. The mean femoral component position was 1.9° externally rotated compared with gap balance (with a variation of 13° internal to 18° external rotation). The femoral rotation was within 3° of gap balancing only 39% of the time.

Finally, the posterior condylar axis produced similar results. The mean rotation of the femoral component was 0.4° internally rotated to the gap balance (with a range of 15° internal rotation to 13° external rotation) The flexion gap wad balanced 58% of the time.

Gap balancing, as described by Insall and colleuages,[2] seems to recreate the flexion gap much more reproducibly than the measured resection techniques. Intuitively this makes sense because all 3 measured resection techniques are static and do not rely on any of the 3 prime determinants of flexion gap symmetry: the tibial resected surface, the MCL complex, and the LCL complex. The 3 measured resection techniques are simple best estimations, based on the femoral anatomy, but they fall short in determining true dynamic balance and flexion symmetry.

Unfortunately, the gap balancing technique remains somewhat subjective and requires years of experience to master. As accurate as this technique is, it does not provide objective data in terms of the compressive forces across the medial and lateral joint lines. This is where the eLibra Dynamic Knee Balancing System has a noted advantage. This device provides real-time data with the use of a force sensor to objectively assess the flexion space and balance the medial and lateral sides by evaluating all 3 prime determinants of the flexion space: the resected tibia, the MCL complex, and the LCL complex (**Fig. 3**).

DESIGN RATIONALE: BALANCED RESECTION

The eLibra Dynamic Knee Balancing system was designed to create objective, real-time data regarding the balance of the medial and lateral ligament complexes in flexion. Through a patented

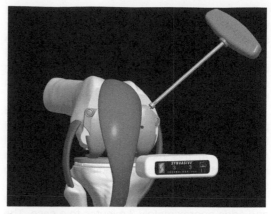

Fig. 3. eLibra Dynamic Knee Balancing System. (*Courtesy of* Zimmer Inc, Warsaw, IN; with permission.)

force sensor device, the eLibra quantifies the compressive forces across the joint in newtons. Each integer on the force sensor represents 15 N of compressive force. These objective real-time data are then used to balance these compressive forces across the joint in flexion prior to the femoral AP bony cuts, allowing surgeons to externally rotate the trial femoral cutting block to the desired balanced rotation. Balanced resection refers to the combination of measured resection and gap balancing. The eLibra creates a balanced flexion space through the use of a measured resection while gap balancing. It eliminates the need for subjective feel of traditional gap balancing measures by providing quantifiable data prior to the resections.

Although gap balancing has been shown in the literature more accurate than measured resection techniques,[22] there are drawbacks to traditional gap balancing:

1. There is no objective feedback with the use of tensiometers or laminar spreaders.
2. The knee joint is not articulated with this technique.
3. Balance is achieved without regard to the patella and the contribution of the lateral patella femoral ligaments.
4. There is no ability to evaluate the flexion space at various degrees of femoral rotation.

The eLibra quantifies soft tissue tension in each compartment, thus eliminating the need for subjective feel. The 3 prime determinants of these compressive forces are the resected tibia and the medial and lateral ligament complexes. The sensor then allows for balancing with both the traditional tibial resection perpendicular to the tibial shaft or the anatomic technique, where the resection is in slight varus.

The knee joint is articulated during balancing with the eLibra and the patella can be reduced or subluxed during balancing. The flexion space can also be evaluated at various degrees of external rotation throughout the maneuver and in varying degrees of knee flexion, although 90° of flexion has been traditionally used for gap balancing.

Optimal balance is then objectively achieved prior to any femoral AP cuts, eliminating the need for any balancing at the end of the case or with trial reduction. In this manner, the device provides intraoperative feedback and adjustability prior to seating of the trial components.

Balancing with the eLibra is simple and intuitive and adds approximately 3 minutes to a case. The technique is easier to learn than traditional gap balancing and has the advantage of providing real-time data, ultimately leading to better flexion gap stability and a symmetric flexion space (**Fig. 4**).

eLibra Dynamic Knee Balancing System Design Specifications

The eLibra system comprises a resterilizable instrument tray (specific to the implant) and a single-use sterile electronic force sensor.

The stainless steel (reusable) eLibra femoral component has a low-profile, implant-like articular

shape that allows for patellar reduction during use. The eLibra femoral component consists of a fixation plate with countersunk holes allowing for temporary fixation by driving screws into the distal femur. This plate is permanently assembled to the articular surface. This assembly contains an adjustment mechanism that allows for 9° of external rotation (relative to the posterior condyles). Adjustment is performed using the supplied torque wrench to turn the adjustment screw located on the anteromedial aspect of the femoral component. The eLibra femoral component contains 3-mm drill holes that correspond to the pin location of the implant 4-in-1 femoral resection guide (**Fig. 5**).

The corresponding eLibra tibial inserts are designed with a dual articular geometry, which allow range of motion from full extension to 90° of flexion prior to AP femoral resections. These inserts are provided in 1-mm increments, ranging from 9 mm to 18 mm (**Fig. 6**).

The eLibra force sensor is a single-use sterile electronic force sensor that measures and displays the relative medial/lateral compartmental forces. This sensor comprises a polymer housing that encapsulates a thick-film sensor element, microprocessor, accelerometer, battery, and an organic light-emitting diode display. During use, an eLibra tibial insert is placed on the sensor; this assembly is then inserted into the joint space between the proximal tibial resection and the eLibra femoral component. Dynamic balance is achieved by externally rotating the lateral condyle

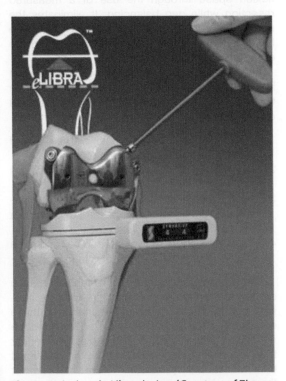

Fig. 4. Articulated eLibra device. (*Courtesy of* Zimmer Inc, Warsaw, IN; with permission.)

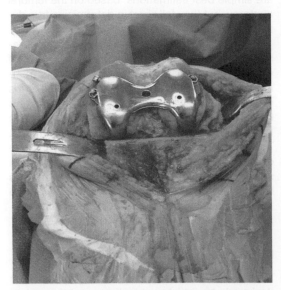

Fig. 5. eLibra femoral trial consisting of trial femur, fixation screws, torque adjustment, and rotation drill holes.

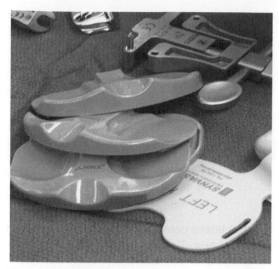

Fig. 6. Trial tibial trays with AP sizer in background.

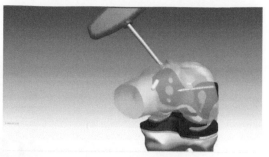

Fig. 8. eLibra photo, posterior transparent view. (*Courtesy of* Zimmer Inc, Warsaw, IN; with permission.)

to contact the trial polyethylene and create a reading on the medial and lateral side of the force sensor (**Figs. 7** and **8**).

ELIBRA SURGICAL TECHNIQUE
Establish Extension Gap by Traditional Methods

The extension gap comprises the distal femoral osteotomy and the proximal tibial osteotomy. This is performed by a surgeon's preferred technique: conventional instrumentation, navigation, or preoperative patient-specific jigs. Extension gap balance then proceeds as usual with

confirmation by extension blocks, ensuring full extension. Alternatively, the eLibra system allows for confirmation of medial lateral balance in extension by use of the appropriate extension paddle and force sensor. These numbers on the force sensor in extension typically are much higher than in flexion because the collaterals are taut in extension and lax in flexion. In addition, the sensor is measuring tension in the posterior capsular structures (**Fig. 9**).

Establish Flexion Gap with eLibra

1. All meniscal remnants and medial or lateral osteophytes are removed prior to placement of the femoral trial because these can tent the collateral ligaments. In addition, every effort should be made to remove posterior osteophytes. Resect the PCL here if performing a cruciate sacrificing knee.
2. The trial femoral component (left or right) is placed onto the distal femur and flush to the posterior condyles. The device is secured to the femur through the use of 2 threaded screws on the superior aspect of the femoral trial. Femoral trial comes in large and small.
3. The force sensor is activated and a tibial trial polyethylene is placed onto the force sensor starting with 10 mm.
4. The sensor is inserted into the knee at approximately 60° of flexion and the knee is then flexed to 90°.
5. Ensure a medial reading that is higher than the lateral reading. The sensor works off a medial pivot design and intact MCL is crucial to proper performance.
6. With the knee flexed at 90°, an assistant elevates the femur slightly and a towel is placed around the Achilles area to elevate the ankle to hold the knee at 90° without any counterforce on the leg from the surgical table. The

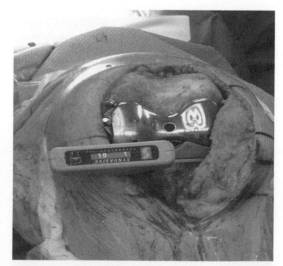

Fig. 7. Assembled femoral trial on force sensor with tibial tray in place. Note higher initial medial force reading at 10 prior to external rotation balancing.

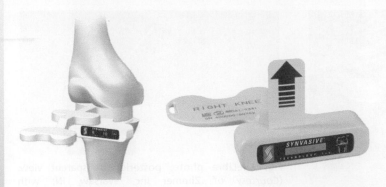

Fig. 9. Optional extension gap measurement. (*Courtesy of* Zimmer Inc, Warsaw, IN; with permission.)

patella is reduced at this stage as well (**Fig. 10**).

7. The anteromedial thumbscrew is turned counterclockwise until the medial and lateral numbers are equal. Optimum balance is in the 3 to 9 range according to manufacturer specifications.

8. Rotation holes are drilled with 3.20-mm drill bit (**Fig. 11**)

9. Femur is sized using knee model–specific sizer with either anterior or posterior referencing, and rotation holes are then used to externally rotate the 4-in-1 cutting jig (**Fig. 12**)

10. Proceed with 4-in-1 distal femoral finishing cuts (**Fig. 13**)

TROUBLESHOOTING WITH THE ELIBRA

Occasionally, the device does not work properly when inserted into the knee. Problems encountered with the device can include the following:

1. Initial lateral compartment force is higher than medial side. This situation is encountered in a tight valgus knee and may require initial lateral side releases in order to balance properly with the eLibra.

2. Force readings never equalize. This situation is encountered with a tight varus knee and requires initial medial collateral releases with an 18-gauge needle or medial subperiosteal stripping.

3. Force readings do not increase despite increasing tibial insert thickness. This situation is encountered with either a lax MCL or when the flexion gap is too large to balance by standard means. The solution to the flexion gap issue is to place a thicker tibial trial with 10-mm augmentation. Then proceed with standard eLibra balancing. A lax MCL is in all likelihood a contraindication for standard eLibra balancing and may require a more constrained prosthesis to make up for an incompetent MCL.

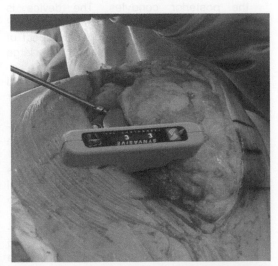

Fig. 10. Force sensor reading equal medial/lateral balance with patella reduced.

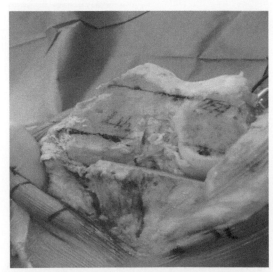

Fig. 11. eLibra line drawn onto femur is bottom line. TEA is the top line drawn for reference.

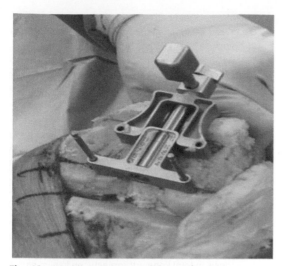

Fig. 12. AP sizing using model-specific sizer.

EARLY CLINICAL RESULTS

Nevins and Leffers[23] describe the use of the eLibra with respect to balancing the MCL in the green zone, defined as the optimum zone at which the MCL is under tension but not too tight as to cause cellular damage. The investigators define this zone as between 9 and 15 kg of force on the medial side. The investigators prospectively followed 50 patients who received a mobile-bearing posterior stabilized knee. The flexion gap was balanced with use of the eLibra. All 50 patients had significant improvements postoperatively in terms of reliance on assistive devices for ambulation and significant decreases in pain scores.

Kreuzer and Leffers[24] describe the use of the eLibra in 50 patients undergoing TKA using

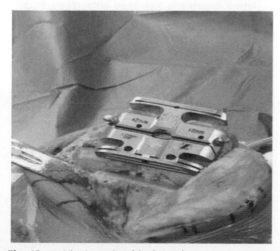

Fig. 13. A 4-in-1 cutting block in place.

navigation for the distal femur and proximal tibia osteotomies and the eLibra for flexion gap balancing. Their results indicate that 30% to 40% of these knees would have had significant flexion instability if traditional measured resection techniques were used to gap balance. These results are similar to published data by Dennis,[14] who found flexion instability in 39% to 58% of cases using traditional measured resection techniques.

Fetto and colleagues[25] found the incidence of lateral retinacular release significantly less with the use of the eLibra; these investigators retrospectively reviewed 100 cases with the eLibra and 100 consecutive cases without the eLibra. The rate of lateral retinacular release with eLibra was 5.5% versus 12% without eLibra.

Finally, De Keyser and Beckers[26] described the effect of patellar subluxation on tibiofemoral pressure distribution in vivo with the use of the eLibra. The investigators studied 32 consecutive patients and found that patellar subluxation increased medial compartmental pressures. After balancing the knee with the patella reduced, there was a significant rise in medial compartment pressures with the patella subluxed (not everted) in all 32 knees. These findings are in contrast to cadaveric studies[27] that describe an increase in lateral pressures with subluxation or eversion of the patella. This finding gives new insight on the role of patellar position during gap balancing in TKA. The eLibra device has led to this insight and will clearly change the way surgeons treat the patella in gap balancing.[28]

SUMMARY

The eLibra Dynamic Knee Balancing System has been proved a helpful surgical tool for use in gap balancing. The device has distinct advantages over traditional gap balancing and measured resection techniques. The device provides objective patient-specific feedback on soft tissue tension to guide femoral rotation before the AP cuts are made. The patella is reduced during balance and the leg is articulated. This allows for balance at various degrees of femoral rotation.

The eLibra quantifies soft tissue tension in each compartment, eliminating subjective feel. Surgeons perform TKA using the balanced resection technique, combining measured resection and precise gap balancing. The instrumentation is a soft tissue preserving technology, sparing unnecessary releases during trial reduction and often accelerating the trial reduction process. The eLibra provides feedback and adjustability prior to committing to femoral resections. In this manner, it allows real-time objective information to dictate the femoral rotation and improve the overall balance of the knee.

REFERENCES

1. Insall J, Tria AJ, Scott WN. The total condylar knee prosthesis: the first 5 years. Clin Orthop Relat Res 1979;145:68–77.
2. Insall JN, Binazzi R, Soudry M, et al. Total knee arthroplasty. Clin Orthop Relat Res 1985;192: 13–22.
3. Sledge CB, Ewald FC. Total knee arthroplasty experience at the Robert breckbrigham hospital. Clin Orthop Relat Res 1979;145:78–84.
4. Sorrells RB. The clinical history and development of the low contact stress total knee arthroplasty. Orthopedics 2002;25(Suppl 2):207–12.
5. Lombardi AV, Berend KR, Adams JB. Patient-specific approach in total knee artthoplasty. Orthopedics 2008;31:1–7.
6. Victor J, Hoste D. Image based computer-assisted total knee arthroplasty leads to lower variability in coronal alignment. Clin Orthop Relat Res 2004; 428:131–9.
7. Dennis DA, Komistek RD, Kim RH, et al. Gap balancing versus measured resection technique for total knee arthoplasty. Clin Orthop Relat Res 2010;468:102–7.
8. Fehring TK, Odum S, Griffin WL, et al. Early failures in total knee arthroplasty. Clin Orthop Relat Res 2001;392:315–8.
9. Krackow KA. Instability in total knee arthroplasty: loose as a goose. J Arthroplasty 2003;18(3 Pt 2): 45–7.
10. Lakstein D, Zarrabian M, Kosashvili Y, et al. Revision totoal knee arthroplasty for component malrotation is highly beneficial: a case control study. J Arthroplasty 2010;7:1047–52.
11. Griffin FM, Insall JN, Scuderi GR. Accuracy of soft tissue balancing in total knee arthroplasty. J Arthroplasty 2010;15(8):970–3.
12. Mihalko WM, Whiteside LA, Krackow KA. Comparison of ligament balancing techniques during total knee arthroplasty. J Bone Joint Surg Am 2003; 85(Suppl 4):132–5.
13. Olcott CW, Scott RD. A comparison of 4 intraoperative methods to determine femoral component rotaton during total knee arthroplasty. J Arthroplasty 2000;15(1):22–6.
14. Dennis DA. Measured resection: an outdated technique in total knee arthroplasty. Orthopedics 2008; 31(9):940, 943–4.
15. Kinzel V, Ledger N, Shakespeare D. Can the Epicondylar axis be defined accurately in Total Knee Arthroplasty. KNEE 2005;12(4):293–6.
16. Yau WP, Leung A, Liu KG, et al. Errors in the identification of the transepicondylar and anteroposterior axes of the distal femur in total knee replacement using minimally-invasive and conventional approaches. J Bone Joint Surg Br 2008;90:520–6.
17. Salvi M, Piu G, Caputo F, et al. Is the 3 degrees external rotation method accurate for the correct rotational alignment of the femoral component in varus knee. J Bone Joint Surg Br 2005;87:200.
18. Middleton FR, Palmer SH. How accurate is Whitesides line as a reference axis in total knee arthroplasty? Knee 2007;14(3):204–7.
19. Yau WP, Chiu KY, Tang WM. How precise is the determination of rotational alignment of the femoral prosthesis in total knee arthroplasty: an in vivo study. J Arthroplasty 2007;22(7):1042–8.
20. Nagamine R, Miura H, Inoue Y, et al. Reliability of the antero-posterior axis and the posterior condylar axis for determining rotational alignment of the femoral component in total knee arthroplasty. J Orthop Sci 1998;3(4):194–8.
21. Fehring TK. Rotational malalignment of the femoral component in total knee arthroplasty. Clin Orthop Relat Res 2000;380:72–9.
22. Lee DH, Park JH, Song DI, et al. Accuracy of soft tissue balancing in TKA: comparison between navigation-assited gap balancing and conventional measured resection. Knee Surg Sports Traumatol Arthrosc 2010;18(3):381–7.
23. Nevins R, Leffers K. Balancing the perfect knee. Podium Presentation ISTA. 2009.
24. Kreuzer S, Leffers K. Soft tissue balance in primary total knee arthroplasties using a force sensing device. ISTA 2009.
25. Fetto J, Hadley S, Schwarzkopf R, et al. Electronic measurement of soft tissue balancing reduces lateral releases in total knee arthroplasty. Podium Presentation at ISTA. 2009.
26. De Keyser W, Beckers L. Influence of patellar subluxation on ligament balancing in total knee arthroplasty through a sub vastus approach. Acta Orthop Belg 2010;76:799–805.
27. Gejo R, McGarry M, Jun B, et al. Biomechanical effects of patellar positioning on intra-operative knee joint gap measurement in total knee arthroplasty. Clin Biomech (Bristol, Avon) 2010;25:353–8.
28. Archibeck MJ, Camarata D, Trauger J, et al. Indications for lateral retinacular release in total knee replacement. Clin Orthop Relat Res 2003;(414):157–61.

Handheld Navigation in Total Knee Arthroplasty

David Mayman, BA, MD

KEYWORDS

- Knee replacement • Computer navigation • Mechanical axis • Tibial alignment • Femora alignment

KEY POINTS

- Knee replacements with tibial malalignment have been shown to lead to higher failure rates.
- A handheld navigation system is accurate and easy to use.
- With price pressure on joint replacement surgery, a disposable unit may be more attractive than an expensive large console system.

INTRODUCTION

Computer navigation for total knee arthroplasty (TKA) has been clinically available for over a decade; yet it remains an uncommonly used technology used today. Multiple clinical studies show that these computerized guides are more accurate than their mechanical counterparts, but they are not used. Several reasons have been sited, including cost, learning curve, additional incisions for pin sites, increased operating room time, line of sight issues, and lack of evidence that clinical outcomes are improved.[1]

The idea of a handheld easy-to-use navigation system was conceived in 2008, and the first system became clinically available in 2009.

Hard parameters were laid down for the development team. These included no additional incisions, no pins in the femur or tibia, no external computer or device that would require line of sight or a nonsterile operator, no capital equipment cost, little to no additional operating room time and a fast learning curve, and accuracy equivalent to or better than currently available large console navigation systems.

There is significant argument in the literature on the clinical need for tools that are more accurate than standard mechanical guides. Many studies show that navigated knee replacements are more likely to be within what is considered appropriate mechanical axis alignment.[2] Several midterm studies have shown no increased failure rates in knees that are not within this accepted alignment, called outliers.[3]

Ritter and colleagues showed increased polyethylene stresses on tibial implants in more than 3° of varus and higher failure rates. They showed a revision rate of 168 for tibias in greater than 3° of varus in patients with a body mass index (BMI) of over 33.[2]

TKA today is done using either a bony resection technique or a ligament-balancing technique. In a ligament-balancing technique, tibial alignment is critical, as femoral rotation is linked to tibial alignment. If the tibial cut is made in 4° of varus, then the femoral implant will be internally rotated by 4°. This may affect patellar tracking and kinematics of the knee.

Current literature shows that 15% to 40% of revision TKAs are done for mechanical loosening. Polyethylene wear and instability are 2 other major reasons for revision. Most remaining revisions are done for infection.[4–8] More precise alignment should decrease the number of failures for mechanical loosening, instability, and polyethylene wear.

Even if outcomes are not improved, every time a surgeon goes into a TKA procedure, the surgeon has a target for alignment in mind. If there is a

The author has nothing to disclose.
Orthopedic Surgery, Hospital for Special Surgery, Cornell University, New York, NY, USA
E-mail address: maymand@hss.edu

Orthop Clin N Am 45 (2014) 185–190
http://dx.doi.org/10.1016/j.ocl.2013.12.002
0030-5898/14/$ – see front matter © 2014 Elsevier Inc. All rights reserved.

simple, easy-to-use tool that allows that target to be hit more frequently, then why would it not be used?

SURGICAL TECHNIQUE

Two systems are currently approved by the US Food and Drug Administration and on the market. These systems are made by OrthAlign (Aliso Viego, California) and Zimmer (Warsaw, Indiana). Both systems work in similar fashion using accelerometer technology. The OrthAlign system surgical technique will be described.

Standard exposure is performed for the knee replacement. Either the distal femoral cut or proximal tibial cut can be performed first.

Distal Femoral Cut

Step 1
The device is pinned to the distal femur with the central pin in the center of the knee. This becomes the center of the knee for the navigation system (**Fig. 1**).

Step 2
An offset adjustment is made for the system to compensate for different sized femurs (**Fig. 2**).

Step 3
The sensors are attached to the mechanical device (**Fig. 3**).

Step 4
The femur is rotated, allowing the system to determine the center of the femoral head (**Fig. 4**).

Step 5
The system now knows the mechanical axis of the femur and shows the current position of the femoral cutting block (**Fig. 5**).

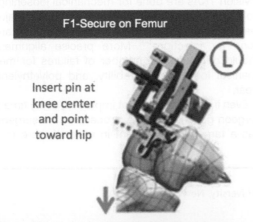

Fig. 1. The device is pinned to the distal femur.

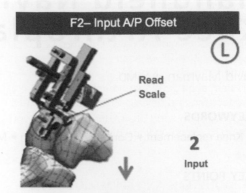

Fig. 2. Offset adjustment is made.

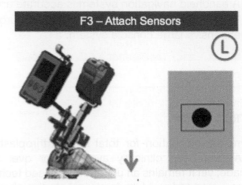

Fig. 3. Sensors are attached to mechanical device.

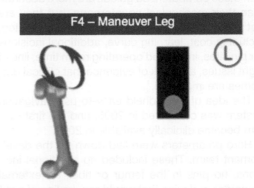

Fig. 4. The femur is rotated.

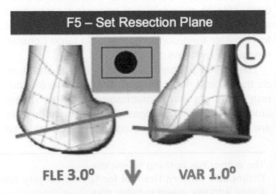

Fig. 5. The system providing a view of the current position of the femoral cutting block.

Step 6
The cutting block is adjusted to the chosen angle using a screw for varus/valgus and a screw for flexion. Real-time numbers are seen for these adjustments. Once alignment of the block has been adjusted, a mechanical stylus is used to set depth of resection. The femoral block is then pinned on the distal femur in the correct position, and the remainder of the device is removed (**Fig. 6**).

Step 7
The distal femoral cut is completed.

Proximal Tibial Cut

Step 1
The tibial device is placed on the tibia with a spring around the midcalf, and 2 short pins are placed in the proximal medial tibia within the incision (**Fig. 7**).

Step 2
The device is centered in the knee, with the stylus sitting on the ACL footprint and the front of the device over the medial third of the tibia (**Figs. 8** and **9**).

Step 3
Offset adjustment is made for the ankle stylus (**Figs. 10** and **11**).

Step 4
Lateral and medial malleoli are registered (**Figs. 12–15**).

Step 5
Alignment is adjusted in real time, and a mechanical stylus is used to measure depth of resection (**Figs. 16–18**).

EVIDENCE

The development and introduction of this device was done in a stepwise fashion with rigorous evaluation.

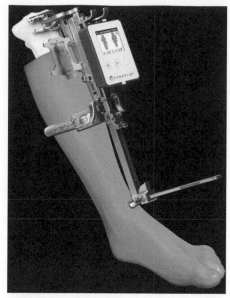
Fig. 7. Placement of the tibial device.

Initial validation of the tibial device was done in a cadaver laboratory study, with cuts evaluated by computed tomography scan. This study showed that mean error from target alignment was 0.68° plus or minus 0.46° for varus/valgus alignment on CT scan. For posterior slope, the mean error was 0.70° plus or minus 0.47°.[9]

The device for the tibia was then evaluated in a single surgeon cohort and a dual surgeon cohort. Tibial alignment was measured on long leg radiographs and showed tibial alignment within 2° of neutral mechanical axis in over 95% of patients.[10,11]

Cadaveric analysis was then performed of the distal femoral device. This showed a mean error of 0.83° plus or minus 0.60° for varus/valgus and 0.83° plus or minus 0.83° for flexion/extension.[12]

Clinical outcomes on the femoral side, again measured with long leg radiographs, showed

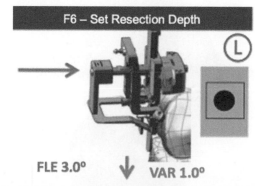
Fig. 6. The cutting block is adjusted to the chosen angle, and then the femoral block is pinned on the distal femur in the correct position.

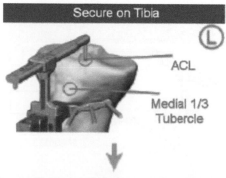
Fig. 8. Centering of device with stylus sitting on ACL footprint.

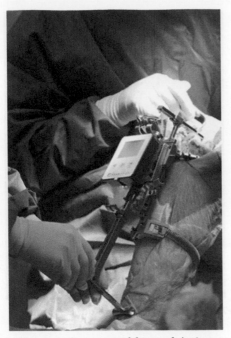

Fig. 9. Showing placement of front of device.

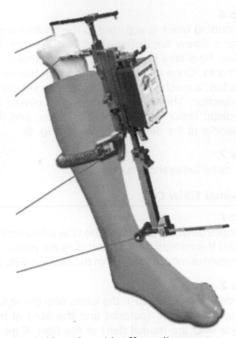

Fig. 11. Ankle stylus with offset adjustment.

95.8% of femoral implants were inserted within 2° of the neutral mechanical axis using the device.[13]

This handheld navigation system has also been compared clinically to a typical large console navigation system. A cohort study was performed comparing 80 knees done with KneeAlign with 80 knees done with AchieveCAS (Orthosoft). This showed that in the Achieve CAS cohort, 86.3% of patients had overall alignment within 3° of neutral mechanical axis compared with 92.5% in the KneeAlign group. Mean tourniquet time was 6 minutes faster with the KneeAlign system than with the Achieve CAS system.[14]

Most recently, a prospective randomized trial was published with multiple surgeons using mechanical guides versus KneeAlign for the tibial cut. This study involving 5 high-volume knee

surgeons showed 95.7% of tibias cut with the KneeAlign system were within 2° of neutral mechanical axis versus 68.1% of knees cut with mechanical guides. Results for posterior slope were similar, with 95.0% of tibias in the KneeAlign group within 2° of target versus 72.1% of tibias cut with mechanical guides.[15]

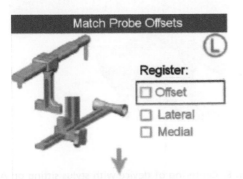

Fig. 10. Offset adjustment is registered.

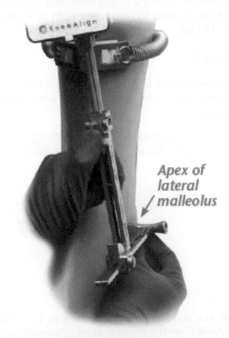

Apex of lateral malleolus

Fig. 12. Apex of lateral malleolus.

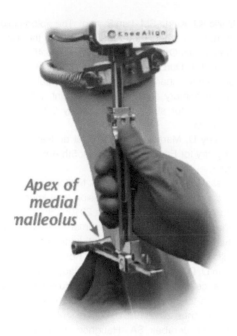

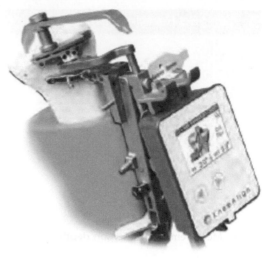

Fig. 16. Placement of device.

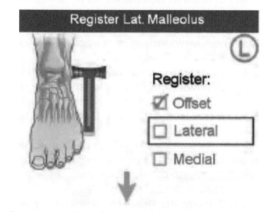

Fig. 13. Apex of medial malleolus.

DISCUSSION

This handheld navigation system clearly allows surgeons to obtain excellent alignment in TKA and has been shown to be equivalent or better than large console navigation systems for alignment. The goals of eliminating capital equipment costs, pin sites, learning curve, increased operative time, and line of sight issues have been addressed.

Surgeons who prefer a ligament balancing technique depend on an accurate tibial cut in order to appropriately balance the knee and end up with an

Fig. 14. Lateral malleolus registered.

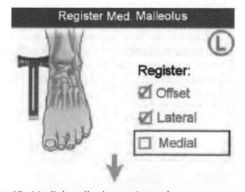

Fig. 15. Medial malleolus registered.

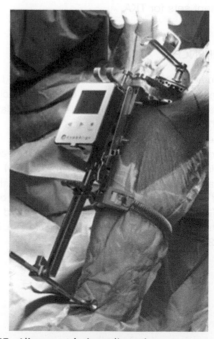

Fig. 17. Alignment being adjusted.

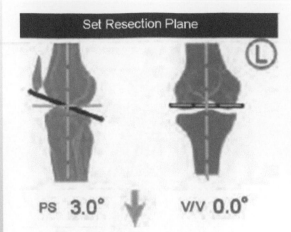

Fig. 18. Measurement of resection depth.

appropriately balanced flexion gap. Surgeons who prefer a bony resection technique depend on accurate tibial and femoral cuts for alignment.

Although there is debate over whether mild amounts of varus lead to early implant failure, there has been increasing discussion of kinematic alignment of the knee where the tibial implant is placed intentionally in slight varus to match the patient's normal anatomy. If this is a technique that is going to be pursued, then a device that allows for accurate measurement and performance of tibial cuts becomes even more critical.

It is likely that as technology continues to improve, handheld smart tools such as this will become more common and part of standard instrument sets for TKA.

REFERENCES

1. Burnett RS, Barrack RL. Computer-assisted total knee arthroplasty is currently of no proven clinical benefit: a systematic review. Clin Orthop Relat Res 2013;471(1):264–76.

2. Berend ME, Ritter MA, Meding JB, et al. Tibial component failure mechanisms in total knee arthroplasty. Clin Orthop Relat Res 2004;428:26–34.

3. Parratte S, Pagnano MW, Trousdale RT, et al. Effect of postoperative mechanical axis alignment on the fifteen-year survival of modern, cemented total knee replacements. J Bone Joint Surg Am 2010; 92(12):2143–9.

4. Bozic KJ, Kuirtz SM, Lau E, et al. The epidemiology of revision total knee arthroplasty in the United States. Clin Orthop Relat Res 2010;468:45–51.

5. Bozic KJ, Durbhakula S, Berry DJ, et al. Different procedure characteristics and hospital resource use in primary and revision total joint arthroplasty: a multicenter study. J Arthroplasty 2005;20(Suppl 3):17–25.

6. Emsley D, Martin J, Newell C, et al. National Joint Registry for England and Wales: 5th Annual Report. 2008.

7. Hossain F, Patel S, Haddad FS. Midterm assessment of causes and results of revision total knee arthroplasty. Clin Orthop Relat Res 2010;468:1221–8.

8. Sharkey PF, Hozack WJ, Rothman RH, et al. Insall Award Paper. Why are total knee arthroplasties failing today? Clin Orthop Relat Res 2001;404:7–13.

9. Nam D, Dy CJ, Cross MB, et al. Cadaveric results of an accelerometer based, extramedullary navigation system for the tibial resection in total knee arthroplasty. Knee 2012;19(5):617–21.

10. Nam D, Jerabek SA, Haughom B, et al. Radiographic analysis of a hand-held surgical navigation system for tibial resection in total knee arthroplasty. J Arthroplasty 2011;26(8):1527–33.

11. Nam D, Cross M, Deshmane P, et al. Radiographic results of an accelerometer-based, handheld surgical navigation system for the tibial resection in total knee arthroplasty. Orthopedics 2011;34(10): e615–21.

12. Nam D, Jerabek SA, Cross MB, et al. Cadaveric analysis of an accelerometer-based portable navigation device for distal femoral cutting block alignment in total knee arthroplasty. Comput Aided Surg 2012;17(4):205–10.

13. Nam D, Nawabi DH, Cross MB, et al. Accelerometer-based computer navigation for performing the distal femoral resection in total knee arthroplasty. J Arthroplasty 2012;27(9):1717–22.

14. Nam D, Weeks KD, Reinhardt KR, et al. Accelerometer-based, portable navigation vs imageless, large-console computer-assisted navigation in total knee arthroplasty: a comparison of radiographic results. J Arthroplasty 2013;28(2):255–61.

15. Nam D, Cody EA, Nguyen JT, et al. Extramedullary guides versus portable, accelerometer-based navigation for tibial alignment in total knee arthroplasty: a randomized, controlled trial: winner of the 2013 HAP PAUL Award. J Arthroplasty 2013. [Epub ahead of print].

Trauma

Trauma

Preface
Trauma

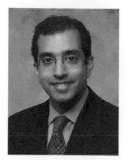

Saqib Rehman, MD
Editor

There are two excellent trauma articles in this issue of the *Orthopedic Clinics of North America* that I hope you will enjoy reading. In our first article, Drs Lowenberg, Githens, and Boone have provided an outstanding, comprehensive review of the principles of tibial fracture management with circular external fixation. Ilizarov techniques and circular fixators continue to be an important tool for the management of orthopedic trauma, particularly in the tibia. However, few surgeons in North America do this as a mainstay treatment in their practice, and many experienced orthopedic trauma surgeons may only do these occasionally. Therefore, it is critical to understand the basic principles of this powerful method. Dr Lowenberg and colleagues have done an excellent job in conveying these principles, and surgeons looking to improve their treatment of tibia fractures will benefit from reading this article.

In our second article, Drs DeBottis, Anavian, and Green review the important topic of surgical management of isolated greater tuberosity fractures of the proximal humerus. These are common injuries and frequently are treated nonoperatively. Shoulder surgeons who sometimes have to manage the sequelae of these injuries have noted that many of these injuries treated nonoperatively would have been better treated surgically. Dr Green has shared his techniques for improving outcomes and the indications for surgical management. I think you will find this article informative if you manage these injuries.

Saqib Rehman, MD
Orthopaedic Surgery
Temple University Hospital
3401 North Broad Street
Philadelphia, PA 19140, USA

E-mail address:
Saqib.rehman@tuhs.temple.edu

http://dx.doi.org/10.1016/j.ocl.2014.01.003
0030-5898/14/$ – see front matter

Principles of Tibial Fracture Management with Circular External Fixation

David W. Lowenberg, MD[a],*, Michael Githens, MD[b],
Christopher Boone, MD[c]

KEYWORDS

- Tibial fracture • Circular external fixation • Llizarov Method • Fine wire fixation
- Multiplanar external fixation

KEY POINTS

- Although circular external fixation is infrequently used for definitive management of tibia fractures, high-energy injuries with significant soft tissue damage and segmental bone loss are well managed with this technique.
- The biomechanical properties of the ring fixator are a result of high-tension transosseous wires allowing for axial micromotion with tremendous coronal and sagittal plane stability.
- In periarticular fractures the articular surface should be reconstructed anatomically by either capsuloligamentotaxis and olive wires or limited internal fixation in combination with wires.
- Frame construction should be based off the metaphyseal reference wire. Olive wires can be used to buttress fracture fragments. Half pins should be used to control and stabilize diaphyseal bone segments. The half pins should be placed in a divergent fashion to further enhance fixation stability.
- A growing body of literature suggests that treatment of high-energy tibial fractures with circular external fixation results in high union rates with limited additional soft tissue complications. There is a lack of long-term studies and quality of life–related outcomes in these patients.

INTRODUCTION AND HISTORY OF EXTERNAL FIXATION FOR FRACTURE MANAGEMENT

Modern fracture care routinely involves the use of external fixation to achieve initial fracture stability with minimal adverse impact on the soft tissues in preparation for definitive management by internal fixation. Although less frequently used, external fixation has an often underappreciated role in definitive management of fractures, both diaphyseal and articular. These injuries are typically high energy in nature, where the soft tissue envelope is in a particularly vulnerable state and must be protected from further insult. Similarly, injuries in which segmental bone loss prevents the use of conventional internal fixation, definitive external fixation with distraction osteogenesis may be used. Although definitive management of fractures with external fixation in the modern era of orthopedic surgery is the exception rather than the rule, methods used today are the result of many years of external fixation development.[1,2]

Although the concept of external fixation had been in use for hundreds of years, Jean Francois Malgaigne, a professor of surgery at University of Paris published advancements in both the concept of indirect fracture reduction and fracture

The authors have nothing to disclose.
a Department of Orthopaedic Surgery, Stanford University School of Medicine, 450 Broadway Street, MC 6342, Redwood City, Stanford, CA 94063, USA; b Department of Orthopaedic Surgery, Stanford University School of Medicine, 450 Broadway Street, MC 6342, Redwood City, Stanford, CA 94063, USA; c Private Practice, Tacoma, Washington, USA
* Corresponding author.
E-mail address: lowenbd@stanford.edu

stabilization through external fixation in the mid 1800s. His device designs, the *pointe métallique* and *griffe métallique,* are considered by many as the forerunners of modern external fixator design.[3]

Surgeons continued to improve on technology and develop new fixators through the nineteenth century, but Clayton Parkhill is credited for the first true uniplanar external fixator. In 1897 he reported on his then novel method of reducing and immobilizing fractures by placing 2 threaded pins above the fracture and 2 below, and connecting them with a set of steel wings and clamps. He went on to publish a series of 14 patients all treated with this method, reporting a 100% rate of union.[3] In 1902 in Antwerp, Belgium, Albin Lambotte reported on a similar unilateral design.[3] These designs were popularized and subsequently improved on through the twentieth century to evolve into what we now know as the unilateral external fixator.

In the mid-1900s, Raoul Hoffman of Geneva, Switzerland, published several articles detailing his design innovations for external fixation, which used adjustable pin-to-bar clamps that, by virtue of sliding up or down the bar, could be used for gross adjustment of fracture angulation and length.[2] His design became the first widely used form of external fixation in North America after the Committee on Fractures and Traumatic Surgery of the American Academy of Orthopedic Surgeons designated it as a useful adjunct to fracture management.[4]

Although unilateral external fixation methods were being improved on throughout Europe and North America in the mid to late twentieth century, developments that would revolutionize our understanding of external fixation from the biomechanics and basic science to deformity, infection, and fracture management were simultaneously under way in Siberia.

The development of circular fixation for the treatment of periarticular and long bone fractures was developed and refined by Gavril A. Ilizarov in Kurgan, Russia. He trained at the Soviet Crimean Medical Institute School of Medicine in Ukraine, and then posted to remote Siberia where he was inundated with many injured World War II veterans. Despite a lack of orthopedic training, Ilizarov treated many war veterans with fractures, malunions, nonunions and infections. As the sole practitioner in a remote and isolated region, improvisation led to innovation and discoveries that are now foundational to our understanding of circular fixation and its wide breadth of applications. His design of crossed fine transosseous wires tensioned to rings above and below a fracture allowed immediate full weight bearing, protecting

against shear forces at the fracture while promoting axial loading at the fracture to enhance healing. It specifically allowed for quicker return of limb function and joint mobilization, which Ilizarov felt was essential to promoting limb healing. Also credited to Dr Ilizarov is the concept of distraction osteogenesis, a discovery that has established a subfield within orthopedic surgery.[2,5]

Most of his work was confined to Siberia until 1968. He then assumed treatment for Valerie Brumel, a national hero and Olympic gold medalist in the high jump who suffered a tibial fracture in a motorcycle accident. He was treated with plate and screw fixation by using early A-O technique and developed an infected nonunion with 2 inches of shortening. On Brumel's return to Moscow after completion of treatment with Ilizarov, he was able to return to competition. Ilizarov and his methods rapidly gained national attention in the Soviet Union. In 1978 he won the Lenin prize for Medicine in the Soviet Union for his work with circular fixation, bone regeneration, and fracture healing.

Ilizarov's method stagnated behind "The Iron Curtain" until 1980 when Carlo Mauri, a famous Italian explorer, learned of Ilizarov's method during his participation in the Ra Expedition. Mauri had suffered a tibial fracture 10 years prior in a mountaineering accident and was left with a nonunion that had failed all conventional treatments. He went to Kurgan and attained full union of his fracture with Ilizarov's method of circular external fixation. This one event opened up the methods of fine wire external fixation to the Western world, as Mauri's physicians from Lecco, Italy, traveled to Kurgan to learn Ilizarov's methods.

In 1982, the Soviet Union opened a hospital dedicated to performing Ilizarov's work in Kurgan. It was a 1000-bed orthopedic hospital, which at that time was the largest orthopedic hospital in the world.

The use of circular external fixation and Ilizarov's methods did not make headway into North America until the later half of the 1980s. A group of surgeons began experimenting with its use in pediatric applications, as well as nonunions, malunions, and limb length inequality. Small groups of American surgeons went to Kurgan in the late 1980s to learn from Ilizarov with the last organized group from America visiting Kurgan in 1989 while the institute was still under Ilizarov's leadership. Ilizarov passed away in 1992. Surgeons throughout the world continue to advance his methods, making it a more conventional mode of fracture management, along with standard techniques of internal fixation. The refined techniques of external fixation are now part of an orthopedic traumatologist's armamentarium. New concepts and designs continue to evolve, enhancing our ability to treat both simple and complex fractures, all while minimizing insult to the soft tissue envelop.

BIOMECHANICS OF CIRCULAR FIXATION VERSUS UNIPLANAR FIXATION

Although the biomechanics of external fixation have been studied substantially, understanding of the mechanical forces across the bone/fixator interface remain poorly understood. To better understand the biomechanical differences between fixator designs, it is instructive to review the evolution of fixator design with each design's historical problems.

The first-generation fixator was a unilateral fixator with the classic "A-frame" design (**Fig. 1**). Although it was effective in stabilizing fractures, there were inherent problems in its use, as not enough emphasis was placed on proper alignment with fragment apposition. A large number of fractures treated with this device went on to nonunion, with the contemporary thinking being the device was excessively rigid. In fact, the fixator was not too rigid; rather, it allowed no axial micromotion while creating excessive shear forces at the fracture site. This lack of axial loading with excessive fracture site shear led to its poor clinical results for definitive fracture care treatment and led to it being labeled a "nonunion maker."

The second generation in fixator design was the unilateral fixator, as we know it today, with the classic prototype being the Hoffman external fixator. Advantages of this design included solid body design in some models, as well as the ease of sliding fixation up and down the stabilization unit. It used parallel half pins above and below a fracture site. These designs gained wide popularity and became the workhorses of external fracture stabilization (**Fig. 2**). Although these fixators worked well for provisional stabilization, they did not provide the proper biomechanical stability necessary to promote appropriate biology for fracture healing. Because of their unilateral design, they were susceptible to shear and torque with axial loading, and displayed significant coronal and sagittal plane bending moment arm to load. This resulted in shear across the fracture site when loading of the limb occurred in any degree of attempted gait. Despite this, it did provide a useful method of fracture stabilization when internal fixation was not appropriate.

The Ilizarov fixator revolutionized concepts of external fixation and represented the third generation in external fixation and was the first to use tensioned fine wires in a multiplanar design. Until then, the merits of multiplanar fixation were overlooked and not appreciated in fracture care (**Fig. 3**). The fine-wire design proved advantageous for fixation of periarticular fractures. It allowed for variable axial micromotion with load modification, such that low loads allow greater

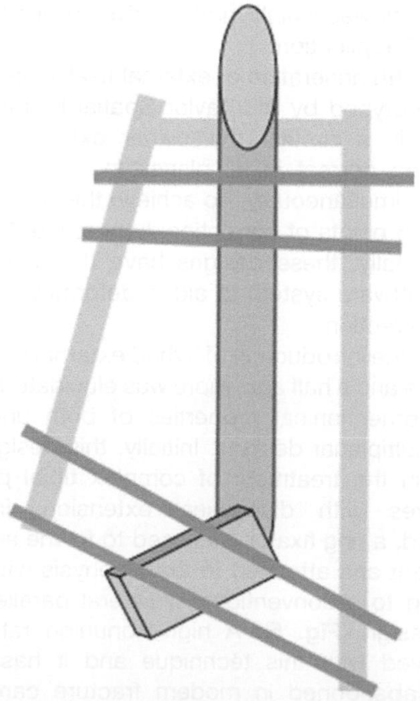

Fig. 1. First-generation "A-frame" external fixator.

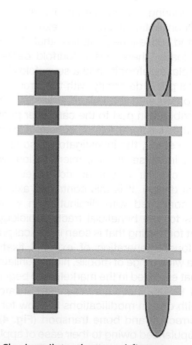

Fig. 2. Classic unilateral external fixator.

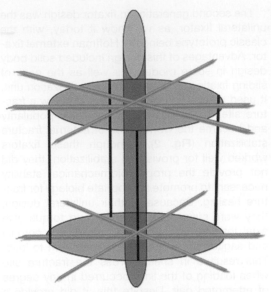

Fig. 3. Schematic of Ilizarov type of external fixation using fine wires under tension and the multiplanar fixation that it resultantly achieved.

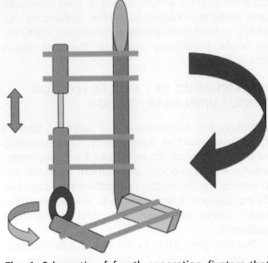

Fig. 4. Schematic of fourth-generation fixators that are unilateral fixators that could deangulate through hinges, as well as lengthen or shorten bone segments in a controlled fashion.

axial motion, and increasing load results in decreasing axial micromotion. This was termed the "trampoline effect," such that increasing load continually tightens the wires and their ability to stretch so that resultant axial deformation exponentially decreases. This axial micromotion in a low shear environment has been shown to be advantageous for callus formation and fracture healing.[6–8]

In comparing multiplanar circular external fixation to conventional uniplanar external fixation, Duda and colleagues[9] found that for similar applied loads, there was a fourfold decrease in coronal plane deformity and a sevenfold decrease in sagittal plane deformity with the circular fixator as compared with the unilateral fixator. This has been attributed in part to the cantilever phenomenon of the unilateral fixator construct design. In this same study, the investigators also showed a 1.75-fold increase in axial micromotion with the fine-wire circular fixator as compared with the unilateral design. It is this controlled axial micromotion combined with diminution in shear that provides for the beneficial fracture biology environment for healing that is seen in clinical practice.

The fourth generation of external fixation includes a wide range of mobile, hinged unilateral fixators that emerged in the marketplace beginning in the mid 1980s. These are essentially unilateral fixators with design modifications to allow for deformity correction and bone transport (**Fig. 4**). They were popularized owing to their ease of application as compared with a circular fixator. These designs,

in essence, are the incorporation of hinges and moving parts into a unilateral, uniplanar fixator.

A fundamental flaw in this generation of fixators is inherent in the basic biomechanical limitations of standard unilateral fixation, principally the excessive shear and bending forces at the fracture site. This led to the limited success of these fixators in clinical practice, particularly in deformity correction and distraction osteogenesis. Their popularity was mainly market-driven owing to their ease of application.

The fifth generation of external fixator are those as prototyped by the Taylor Spatial Frame. This fixator is a circular multiplanar external fixator that can correct in all planes in 3-dimensional space simultaneously. To achieve this, the design allows 6 points of correction; hence, the 6 struts. Additionally, these designs have the advantage of a software system to aid in deformity analysis and correction.

With the introduction of hybrid external fixation a decade and a half ago, more was elucidated about the biomechanical properties of both unilateral and multiplanar designs. Initially, this design was used in the treatment of complex tibial plateau fractures with diaphyseal extension. In this method, a ring fixator was used to fix the articular segment and attached to the diaphysis with bars leading to a conventional unilateral parallel half-pin design (**Fig. 5**). A high nonunion rate was observed with this technique and it has since been abandoned in modern fracture care. The additive effect of 2 distinct attributes of each

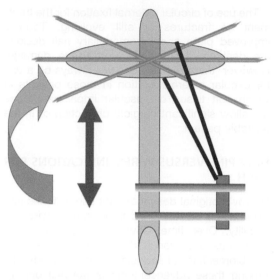

Fig. 5. Schematic of hybrid external fixation. This led to exaggerated shear due to the axial micromotion of the fine wire fixation combined with the torque and shear from the unilateral shaft component of fixation.

form of external fixation at the 2 fixation blocks is responsible for its failure. At the diaphyseal level, unilateral fixation generates higher shear forces and torque. At the epiphyseal/metaphyseal level, fine wire fixation allows for higher axial micromotion. This axial micromotion magnifies the shear and torque seen at the fracture site from the unilateral fixation, creating an unfavorable environment for fracture healing.

With regard to biomechanical stability of circular external fixation, Lowenberg and colleagues[10] showed that the fracture obliquity has a direct bearing on the overall bone-frame construct stability. They found that progressive fracture obliquity led to greater shear. They concluded that fracture obliquity over 30° led to shear becoming a dominant factor with physiologic fracture loading. This could be modified with changes in frame construction and design by adding additional forms of fixation to include arced wires and steerage pins. Lenarz and colleagues,[11] in the same journal, found that the incorporation of 3 divergent half pins for diaphyseal fixation, with divergence angles at 60° in 3-dimensional space, was at least as stable and resistant to shear as any other more involved fixation construct. This information has helped changed the way fixation is performed in the tibia.

INDICATIONS FOR CIRCULAR EX FIX VERSUS INTERNAL FIXATION METHODS

Although modern techniques and implant design continue to improve, there still remains a subset

of fractures that are more amenable to definitive treatment with external fixation devices. General factors to consider when evaluating the use of internal fixation methods versus circular external fixation as definitive management include (1) overall risk/benefit of each method, (2) surgeon experience and training, and (3) the ability to predict and treat possible complications of the selected method. One must also not forget that psychological tolerance and compliance are vastly different from patient to patient and must not be left out of the decision-making process.[12]

Although indications and use of circular external fixation differ from surgeon to surgeon, all would agree that the use of these devices is best in high-energy lower extremity injuries with significant bone loss or soft tissue compromise.[3,13–15]

These complex injuries are often devoid of significant soft tissue, making soft tissue dissection for internal fixation a problem.[3]

A review of the literature reveals extensive support for circular external fixation for intra-articular and extra-articular fractures of the tibia. The tibial soft tissue sleeve is limited and often disrupted in high-energy injuries. There is often also significant segmental bone loss in these injuries. Circular fixation devices or even minimal internal fixation with circular frames have been shown to provide adequate outcomes in these problem fracture patterns. In cases of significant diaphyseal bone loss, circular frames can be used to provide initial shortening and soft tissue closure with the plan to later restore length through distraction osteogenesis.[16] This technique was described by Ilizarov[17] in 1969, and Green[18] and colleagues found relatively good outcomes in patients treated with this method. Of the 17 patients treated, Green and colleagues had union rate of 94%. They did note, however, that this technique is not without its complications; most commonly wire site infections and frame loosening. Although wire site infection continues to pose a problem, frame loosening is no longer an issue because of our better understanding of the technique. Six patients in this series also required late bone-grafting procedures. Overall, there were no long-term nerve or vessel complications and outcomes for this difficult problem were acceptable. Although complications do exist, circular external fixation with distraction osteogenesis remains a powerful tool for treatment of complicated tibial bone defect injuries.[17,18]

Although improved implant design, specifically locked plating, has led to improved outcomes of short-segment articular fractures, circular fixators also have been shown to be a powerful tool in treating these fractures. Watson and Coufal[19] showed good results when applying external fixation devices in combination with minimal internal fixation in high-energy atypical tibial plateau fractures. At follow-up, all 14 complex fractures had healed and 85% had good or excellent Knee Society clinical rating scores. Watson[19] and colleagues felt that this combined method showed excellent clinical results without the severe soft tissue complications often seen with extensive surgical exposure and internal fixation. Using the same principle Raikin and Froimson[20] also found 82% excellent or good outcomes on the Knee Society clinical ratings scale. It should, however, be noted that both investigators recognized that this technique is not without complications. Both listed multiple surgeries, delayed union, delayed bone grafting, pin tract infections, and difficulty with patient hygiene as common occurrences. Krupp and colleagues[21] recently published results on treatment of bicondylar tibial plateau fractures using locked plating versus external fixation. Overall, they found average time to union was 6 months for the locked plating group versus 7 months for the external fixation group. Knee stiffness and malunion were significantly higher in the group treated with ringed external fixation. Even in the face of this new technology, Krupp and colleagues[21] felt that use of circular external fixation for tibial plateau fractures was still a viable option in cases of severe soft tissue injury or comminution, as well as in the unstable patient.

For much the same reasons as the proximal tibia, distal tibial fractures also have been treated with circular external fixation devices. Again the soft tissue envelope around the distal tibia is scant and surgical dissection of injuries with already present soft tissue injury is fraught with complications. Raikin and Froimson[20] described the outcomes of these injuries when treated with circular fixators. They found a 90% rate of union at an average of 4.8 months (n = 20). They reported 3 superficial and 2 deep infections and found post healing ankle range of motion averaged 5° of dorsi flexion and 26° of plantar flexion. All patients recovered at least neutral ankle flexion after frame removal and physical therapy. Overall, they reported a 70% excellent or good outcome when treating these difficult fractures with circular external fixation.

Circular external fixation has also been described in the treatment of femoral shaft as well as upper extremity injuries. Most would agree that internal fixation is likely the modality of choice in these locations; however, one should not exclude from their armamentarium external fixation in these locations, especially in the face of severe soft tissue compromise or in the unstable patient.

The use of circular external fixation for the treatment of fractures is still evolving. Today's improved plate and intramedullary nail designs are designed for minimal soft tissue damage. However, there remains and will always be a use for circular external fixation in those patients in which soft tissue or vascular impairment does not allow significant surgical dissection or in the unstable patient.

HALF PINS VERSUS WIRES, INDICATIONS FOR EACH

Ilizarov's original design did not use half pins and relied solely on tensioned transosseous wires for stability. Over time, advancements have been made based on longitudinal clinical experience and biomechanical analysis of various constructs. Among these advancements is the half pin, intended to stably fix a bony segment to the ring construct while not tying up soft tissue, as is the case with wire fixation.

Although Ilizarov's original design achieved tremendous coronal, sagittal, and torsional stability, it came at the cost of requiring many wires in multiple planes. A maximally stable construct required four levels of fixation for each bone segment, 2 proximally and 2 distally, with 2 crossing wires at each level. The transfixion wires traverse skin, subcutaneous tissues, facial places, and muscle, and as such, can be a source of pain and limitation in motion for the patients, particularly with activation of the muscle groups through which these pins pass during weight bearing. Similarly, as the number of transosseous wires increases, so does the risk of pin-related complications, most notable of which is pin site infection.

A group of Italian surgeons applying Ilizarov's methods in the early 1980s recognized the morbidity associated with wire transfixion of soft tissues, particularly with the anterior to posterior proximal femoral wire. They began substituting a half pin for this wire, finding it to be less morbid yet sufficiently stable.[22,23] Stuart Green and his colleagues[24] noted similar soft tissue–related morbidity and pin site complications in their early cohort treated with circular external fixation and over time began replacing infected wires with titanium half pins mounted to the ring. In a preliminary report comparing patients with traditional wire-only constructs to a cohort with hybrid wire and half-pin constructs, the half pin group had fewer pin site infections, less pain, better motion, and lower surgical time compared with the traditional design. This work paved the way for development of combined wire and half-pin fixation in North America.

Diaphyseal half pins have the obvious advantage of stable fixation with minimal soft tissue transfixion. Pin placement is generally safer and faster, and simplifies the frame application. Biomechanical studies have shown that adequate stability can be maintained with substitution of half pins for wires. Calhoun and colleagues[25] showed that the rigidity of a single tensioned wire is achieved with 2 half pins.

In the tibia, a combination of tensioned transfixion wires and half pins should be used for frame construction, adhering to proper indications of both. Tensioned wires should be used in periarticular segments and metaphyseal bone. The periarticular reference rings should be fixed with a metaphyseal reference wire first rather than a half pin. Wires are useful in controlling small bony segments, and olive wires can be used to gain greater control over segments by buttressing in different vectors. Half pins may be used in meta-diaphyseal and diaphyseal bone to reduce the number of wires needed. They should be off axis to corresponding wire planes for enhanced stability and placed in a divergent manner. Roberts and colleagues[26] demonstrated significantly enhanced construct stability by adding an anterior juxta-articular half pin when treating proximal tibia fractures with circular external fixation.

There is evidence to suggest that use of hydroxyapatite (HA)-coated half pins may reduce pin site infections and enhance pull out strength when used in place of noncoated equivalents.[27] Most North American surgeons have converted to the use of HA-coated half pins when placing a circular fixator with the intent of leaving on an individual for any extended length of time.

The exact combination of wires and pins varies based on surgeon preference, pathology treated, and anatomic considerations. Although Ilizarov's design used 4 rings with 2 wires on each ring for adequate segment control of a fracture, many experts in the field can now achieve adequate stability with a single ring per fixation level. All of Ilizarov's principles still apply with this modification in technique, it is just the methods of fixation that have changed. The proper use of divergent half pins, and addition of extra divergent wires on a ring, as well as the combination of wires and half pins to a fixation segment have allowed for this to be successfully accomplished.

REVIEW OF PUBLISHED CLINICAL RESULTS
Plateau

Early treatment of high-energy tibial plateau fractures by means of open reduction and internal fixation was fraught with a high complication rate.[28–30] An already traumatized soft tissue envelop, subject to further iatrogenic insult, was the principal source of this, with infection and soft tissue complications of 20% reported in early series but approaching 80% in some. Early series reporting results after treatment of similar injuries with the Ilizarov method were promising, although limited to small retrospective cohorts.[31–33] Although underpowered and subject to much bias, these studies reported lower infection and soft tissue complication rates, and promoted the benefits associated with immediate weight bearing including improved Knee Society Scores and range of motion.[31–33] Encouraging early results paved the way for further use of this technique and promoted improved clinical study design.

Mikulak and colleagues[34] retrospectively reviewed 24 patients with Schatzker VI tibial plateau fractures treated with fine wire external fixation and corroborated earlier studies' findings of high union rates with minimal soft tissue trauma, low rates of infection, and good functional outcomes.

Although much emphasis had been placed on the benefits of minimal soft tissue trauma and early weight bearing in these studies, fracture reduction quality and its impact on outcomes had been overlooked. Kumar and Whittle[35] retrospectively reviewed 57 patients with Schatzker VI injuries, evaluating reduction quality and functional outcomes. They found that although all injuries went on to union, 45 anatomically united fractures had a mean Knee Society Score of 83, whereas 9 nonanatomic fracture reductions went on to a mean Knee Society Score of 52. The investigators note that patients who underwent limited open reduction of the articular surface under direct visualization had anatomic reductions and higher Knee Society Scores than those who did not. The investigators concluded that although the Ilizarov method is an acceptable treatment option, it must be accompanied by a limited open approach with anatomic restoration of the articular surface for any injury with articular depression so as to maximize functional outcomes.[35]

Limited internal fixation in concert with circular external fixation has emerged over time as an effective treatment option for bicondylar proximal tibia fractures.[36–38] The Canadian Orthopedic Trauma Society performed a multicentered prospective randomized controlled trial comparing results of open reduction internal fixation (ORIF) (n = 23, nonlocked medial and lateral constructs) with limited internal fixation and circular external fixation (n = 29) for bicondylar tibial plateau fractures. Patients treated with external fixation had shorter hospital stays, faster return to function, and lower complication rates. Clinical outcomes were similar and reduction quality was no different between groups, although the rate and severity of complications was much higher in the ORIF group. For these reasons, the investigators concluded that circular external fixation with limited internal fixation is an attractive treatment modality for bicondylar tibial plateau fractures.[36] This is especially true for those bicondylar fractures with significant shaft comminution and/or extension.

Krupp and colleagues[21] reported conflicting results when they retrospectively compared demographically similar groups of patients with bicondylar injuries treated with either ORIF with locked constructs (n = 30) or circular external fixation (n = 28). The group treated with ORIF had decreased time to union (5.9 vs 7.4 months), decreased incidence of articular malunion (7% vs 40%), better knee motion, and fewer complications (27% vs 48%). Of note, only 2 of the 28 patients in the external fixator group underwent limited internal fixation at the articular surface, again highlighting the need for proper reduction and the role of limited internal fixation to achieve improved articular reduction.

Mahadeva and colleagues[39] performed a systematic review evaluating the published literature on treatment of bicondylar tibial plateau fractures with hybrid external fixation and concluded that circular frames with limited internal fixation have superior clinical results, although the overall quality of literature is weak. The investigators indicate a lack of long-term follow-up in these patients and emphasize that although improved knowledge of soft tissue handling has decreased complication rates, they are still high and current treatment methods leave room for improvement.

Although most high-energy tibial plateau fractures treated with circular external fixation are bicondylar patterns, the benefits of the Ilizarov method can be applied to unicondylar injuries as well. Watson and Coufal[19] retrospectively reviewed the results of 14 high-energy Schatzker Type I and II fractures treated with limited internal fixation and circular external fixation. All patients achieved fracture union although one patient experienced loss of articular reduction and mechanical axis deviation at 6 months. None returned to the operating room for wound-related complications. One patient developed wound slough managed conservatively and a total of 5 infected wires were removed in clinic. There were no deep infections. Functional outcomes were good to excellent in most patients, with 11 of 14 returning to preinjury work status.[19] The investigators note that this cohort represents an atypical variant of the Schatzker I-II injury in which high energy has

been imparted to the soft tissues and, for these, a combined limited internal fixation and Ilizarov construct can afford excellent outcomes.

More recently, Ramos and colleagues[40] have reported prospectively on a cohort of unicondylar and bicondylar plateau fractures treated with classic Ilizarov fixation technique. Eleven patients were treated for Schatzker type I-IV injuries and 19 for Schatzker type V-VI injuries, including both high-energy and low-energy mechanisms in both cohorts. All patients were managed with the same postoperative protocol. All went on to union. Unicondylar fractures had shorter operative time, better knee range of motion, and better subjective outcome scores. Two patients required return to the operating room for debridement of infected pin sites and 2 patients eventually underwent total knee arthroplasty. No arthrotomies for direct articular fracture visualization were done and no fractures were treated with limited internal fixation. The investigators conclude that the Ilizarov method is a valuable treatment method for tibial plateau fractures of all types.[40]

Diaphyseal/Segmental

Literature regarding treatment of diaphyseal tibia fractures with the Ilizarov method is heavily weighted toward the use of bone transport for posttraumatic segmental defects and management of osteomyelitis. Less has been focused on early definitive management of shaft fractures with circular frames. In 1992, Tucker and colleagues[41] reviewed the outcomes of 26 open diaphyseal fractures without segmental bone loss after treatment with a standard Ilizarov frame. All went on to unite without bone grafting, a result not achieved with conventional plating or intramedullary (IM) nailing at the time. There was one case of deep infection related to a wire site requiring debridement and no infections at the site of open fracture. Malunion occurred in 19% of these patients, notably higher than subsequent studies. Operative time decreased from 3.5 hours to 90 minutes as the investigators developed a frame application protocol.[41] The high rate of malunion is clearly not within our current standards of acceptable fracture management.

More recently, El-Sayed and Atef[42] evaluated the role of small wire external fixation for low-energy simple diaphyseal fractures. A total of 324 patients underwent circular frame application and percutaneous lag screw augmentation when possible. All went on to union with no delayed union and maintained excellent knee and ankle motion. Only minor complications were encountered, but pin site infections occurred in 25% of patients. The investigators concluded that although this method is successful for establishing union, it can be expensive, technically challenging, and more difficult for patients postoperatively than IM nailing. The benefits of the Ilizarov method are marginal in simple closed diaphyseal tibia fractures and IM nailing remains the standard treatment.

Circular external fixation has been used with success in early definitive treatment of high-energy open and segmental tibial shaft fractures. Multiple groups have reported a 100% union rate.[14,43,44] Other series report a union rate of 90% to 92%.[13,45,46] Nonunion rates for IM nailing of open and segmental tibia fractures vary from 3% to 22%. A clear advantage of the Ilizarov method over IM nailing is the versatility of managing large bone defects with biconfocal distraction-compression or distraction osteogenesis alone, as well as deformity correction postoperatively with frame adjustment.[47,48] Malunion in recent studies is an infrequently reported complication, whereas pin and wire related complications vary widely and approach 48% in some series.[47]

Inan and colleagues[49] compared the radiographic results and clinical outcomes of unreamed tibial nailing (IMN) and Ilizarov external fixation for the treatment of type IIIA open injuries. Sixty-one patients with open type IIIA tibial shaft fractures were treated with the Ilizarov method (n = 32) or IMN (n = 29). The average time to union was significantly shorter in the Ilizarov group (P = .039). There was no difference in the rate of malunion. Posttraumatic osteomyelitis occurred in 2 patients in the Ilizarov group and in 3 patients in the nailing group. Three patients treated with external fixation returned to the operating room: 1 for sequestrectomy, and 2 for pin exchange. In the IMN group, 7 patients needed additional surgery, including bone grafting (n = 3), nail exchange (n = 1), and posttraumatic osteomyelitis (n = 3). To our knowledge, this is the only study to directly compare circular external fixation and IMN for high-energy open tibial shaft fractures.[49] Although it is retrospective in nature, it seems to confirm a higher rate of nonunion and delayed union and a trend toward higher rates of posttraumatic osteomyelitis at the fracture site after IMN. Long-term and well-designed randomized controlled trials in this area are lacking.

Pilon

Intra-articular fractures of the tibial plafond are notoriously difficult injuries to treat, and the higher-injury more comminuted fracture patterns generally have a poorer long-term functional outcome regardless of the treatment method used. When the talus is driven into the plafond, a tremendous amount of energy is imparted to the articular surface, resulting in severe chondral damage, comminution of the articular and metaphyseal bone, and significant soft tissue injury. Attempts at early internal fixation failed spectacularly in the high-energy injury group, with high rates of wound complications and infection.[50] A staged protocol with early external fixation followed by definitive internal fixation after the soft tissues have recovered was developed with a dramatic decrease in rates of wound problems and deep infection.[51] Alternatively, circular external fixation with limited open reduction of the articular surface and limited internal fixation has become an increasingly attractive treatment for these injuries.

Lovisetti and colleagues[52] combined circular external fixation and limited internal fixation for management of 30 Orthopaedic Trauma Association (OTA) type C pilon fractures and achieved a 100% rate of union. They achieved an anatomic reduction in only 5, good in 23, and fair in 2. Clinical outcomes were similarly spread, with only 6 patients achieving excellent outcome, 9 good, 13 fair, and 2 poor. There were no wound complications or deep infections. Prior series evaluating limited internal fixation in concert with external fixation achieved similarly low infection rates and soft tissue complications.[53–55] In their series, Tornetta and colleagues[55] were able to achieve an anatomic reduction in 36 of 37 pilon fractures, although more internal fixation was used in their series than that of Lovisetti and colleagues.[52] Despite these encouraging results, others have reported nonunion rates of 16% to 21%,[56,57] osteomyelitis in more than 20% of patients, and poor functional outcomes.[57]

In a retrospective comparison of OTA type C pilon fractures treated with either staged ORIF or hybrid fixation, Bacon and colleagues[57] found no significant difference in rates of union, malunion, or infection. They noted a slower time to union in the ORIF group. To date, no well-designed randomized controlled trails have compared circular external fixation to ORIF for these injuries. Although most of the literature is retrospective in nature, there seems to be evidence to support the use of circular external fixation with limited internal fixation for these injuries, and possibly a trend toward improved union rates and less posttraumatic osteomyelitis. Despite these potential benefits, functional outcomes are variable, with many patients suffering long-term sequelae of these injuries despite the treatment offered.

The use of ankle-spanning constructs to capitalize on capsuloligamentotaxis for fracture reduction is controversial. Some argue that spanning the ankle leads to long-term stiffness and deprives the articular cartilage of important nutrients by limiting hydrostatic pressure in the joint. Proponents of the technique argue that spanning the joint is required at least initially to aid in and hold near anatomic reduction. As of now there is currently no consensus in the literature as to which injuries respond best to ankle-spanning constructs and for what length of time the ankle should be immobilized or spanned.[57–60] A primary criticism of spanning the ankle is resultant stiffness. Kapoor and colleagues[58] achieved 10° of dorsiflexion in 75% of their cohort after removing the foot mounting at 3.7 weeks. Kim and colleagues[59] removed their foot mounting after 6 to 10 weeks and achieved good functional recovery in 71% of patients. Some advocates of this technique argue that loss of tibiotalar motion does not correlate with functional disability in these patients. It has become clearer that it is advantageous to span the ankle if there is a risk for ensuing equinus due to soft tissue contracture after a free tissue transfer about the distal leg or ankle, or if the patient has impairment of ankle dorsiflexion. Lowenberg and colleagues[61] showed improved functional results with temporary ankle spanning in such a patient population subset.

CASE EXAMPLE

A 35-year-old man fell from 12 feet off a ladder while working, landing on his left foot. He was taken to the hospital, and workup revealed an isolated closed left tibial pylon fracture and distal fibular shaft fracture. He was treated by the on-call orthopedic surgeon with plating of his fibula and placement of a spanning tibial-calcaneal unilateral fixator (**Fig. 6**). A computed tomography scan was then performed to further delineate the fracture (**Fig. 7**).

On postoperative day 1, the patient developed moderate fracture blisters around his ankle and was transferred for a higher level of care.

The patient was treated with leg elevation, and after 7 days the swelling had decreased. The soft tissue envelope was still quite compromised due to the degree and extent of fracture blisters. It was therefore determined that limited ORIF of the joint surface in conjunction with circular external fixation for the metaphyseal/diaphyseal extension would be the most optimal treatment. He was then taken to the operating room for limited internal fixation of the articular components of the fracture, and placement of a circular fixator to bridge the epiphyseal/metaphyseal segment to the diaphysis (**Fig. 8**).

The patient did well following surgery and was kept non–weight bearing, but allowed immediate ankle motion. Specific attention was given to maintaining a plantigrade foot, and ensuring that at least 5° ankle dorsiflexion was present. Radiographs taken 6 weeks postoperative show maintenance of reduction and alignment and early healing (**Fig. 9**).

At 3 months postoperative, weight bearing was initiated, and at 4 months, the fixator was removed

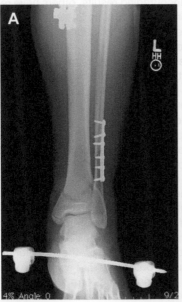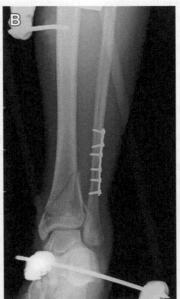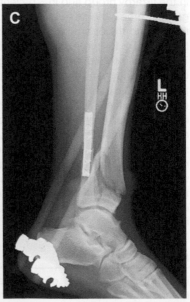

Fig. 6. Anteroposterior (AP) (*A*), mortise (*B*), and lateral (*C*) of left ankle following plating of fibula and spanning external fixation.

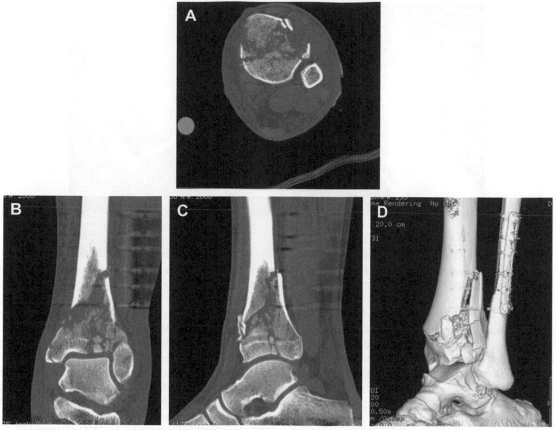

Fig. 7. (*A–D*) Computed tomography scan with reformations of left ankle. Note the severe comminution of the anterolateral column.

with the fracture healed (**Fig. 10**). The patient was backed down to limited weight bearing, then advanced to full weight bearing again over 4 weeks.

The patient did well and rapidly returned to full activities, including playing golf for recreation. He had occasional discomfort requiring over-the-counter NSAIDs for the first several months.

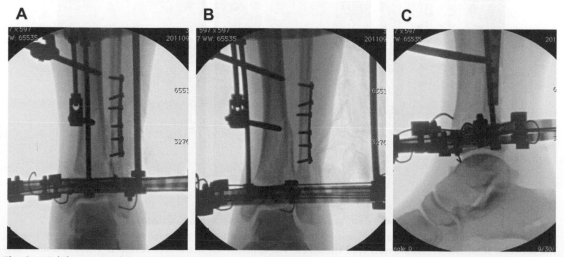

Fig. 8. AP (*A*), mortise (*B*), and lateral view (*C*) intraoperatively. The joint surface and alignment are restored.

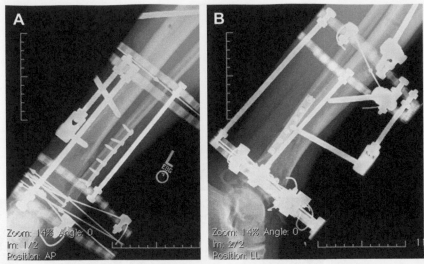

Fig. 9. AP (*A*) and lateral view (*B*) of distal tibia in fixator. The metaphyseal/diaphyseal junction is showing early evidence of healing. The patient is freely ranging his ankle with a plantigrade foot.

At the 1-year postsurgical repair follow-up visit, he had a normal gait pattern with no real limitation in activities. He had 5° less dorsiflexion than on the contralateral side. He took no analgesics and could walk a full golf course while playing golf (**Fig. 11**).

DISCUSSION

Circular external fixation is a valuable tool in the orthopedic traumatologist's armamentarium for treatment of long bone fractures, both articular and diaphyseal. Although frame application can be technically challenging, a sound understanding of the frame's biomechanical principles, and techniques for specific indications, will bring clarity to the process. Careful and thoughtful preoperative planning, proper frame application, and patient selection with appropriate postoperative monitoring are all critical to successful treatment.

Use of the Ilizarov method for fracture management in the tibia has distinct advantages over other

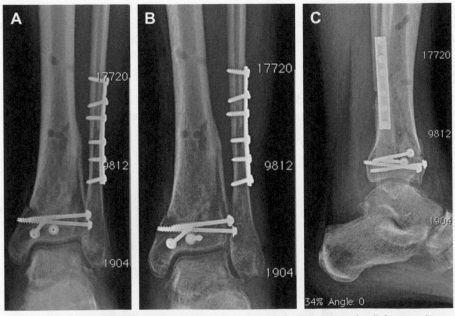

Fig. 10. AP (*A*), mortise (*B*), and lateral view (*C*) following circular fixator removal. All fracture lines are healed. The articular segment screws are now well visualized. The articular surface is well restored. There is disuse osteoporosis seen across the joint and hindfoot.

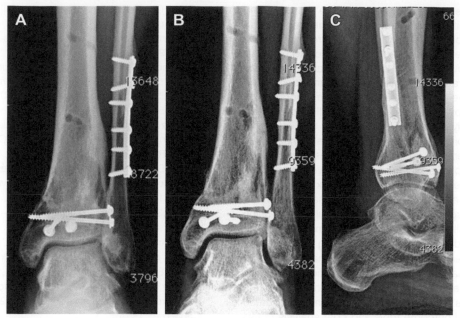

Fig. 11. AP (*A*), mortise (*B*), and lateral view (*C*) 1 year following surgical repair. The joint is preserved with good bone alignment.

modalities for specific injury patterns but is not intended to treat all fractures. Low-energy injuries with little soft tissue insult are typically well managed by internal fixation with low risk to the soft tissue envelope. Conversely, there is a clear role for circular external fixation in high-energy injuries in which there may be significant soft tissue injury or segmental bone loss.

When applying a circular external fixator, the surgeon must understand the concepts of properly balancing the fixator in an orthogonal fashion on the limb. He must also understand the need for obtaining appropriate fracture and limb stabilization at each fixation block. He must also properly reduce the fracture either with direct reduction at the articular segments or indirect reduction using the fixator itself or via a host of other techniques. The need for limited internal fixation at an articular surface is usually an essential part of the treatment. The fixator cannot make up for poor technique or poor reduction.

Management of articular fractures, both at the plateau and plafond, should be treated with anatomic restoration of the articular surface, either by direct reduction and limited internal fixation, or by capsuloligamentotaxis, followed by meta-diaphyseal stabilization with circular external fixation. Olive wires should be used to control and buttress small fragments where possible. Half pins should be used in the diaphysis to minimize soft tissue transfixion and reduce the number of fine wires needed. Implant design and surgical technique have improved the outcomes of these difficult fractures over that past 20 years; however, ringed external fixation with or without minimal internal fixation will often be required in cases in which the soft tissues are significantly compromised.

Our understanding of outcomes after treatment of tibial fractures with circular external fixation is based largely on small retrospective analyses with short-term follow-up. Much effort has been invested in understanding perioperative complication rates and union rates, whereas there is a relative paucity of data on patient satisfaction and objective functional outcomes. Patients who sustain these injury patterns often have multiple other traumatic injuries, varying medical comorbidities, and variable demographic profiles making well-controlled randomized trials with long-term follow-up very difficult to perform. To our knowledge, there is only one article addressing long-term outcome and cost of tibial limb salvage versus amputation using circular fixation, bone transport, and free tissue transfer. Lowenberg and colleagues[62] published a series of 34 such patients with a mean and medial follow-up of 11 years. Their results showed a cost savings with low long-term reintervention rate and good functional outcome. Clearly, more such studies are needed.

Despite these challenges, there is a growing mass of literature to suggest that circular external fixation for high-energy tibial fractures has advantages over traditional internal fixation with potential improved rates of union, decreased incidence of posttraumatic osteomyelitis, and decreased soft tissue problems. The Ilizarov method comes with its own unique set of complications, most commonly being pin site irritation and infection. Frame construction can be technically challenging and expensive, and the patient must be willing to actively participate in postoperative frame care. When the principles of circular external fixation are properly applied, definitive management of high-energy tibia fractures can result in high union rates while minimizing severe complications. To further advance our understanding of the role of circular external fixation in the management of these tibial fractures, randomized controlled trials should be implemented. In addition to complication rates and radiographic outcomes, validated functional outcome tools and cost analysis of this method should be compared with open reduction with internal fixation.

REFERENCES

1. Hippocrates. Works of Hippocrates. Baltimore (MD): Williams & Wilkins; 1946.

2. LaBianco GJ, Vito GR, Rush SM. External fixation. In: Southerland J, Alder D, et al, editors. McGlamry's comprehensive textbook of foot and ankle surgery, vol. 1, 3rd edition. Philadelphia: Lippincott, Williams & Wilkins; 2001. p. 107–8.

3. Browner B, Levine A, Jupiter J, et al. Skeletal trauma. 2nd edition. Philadelphia: WB Saunders; 1998.

4. Klapp F. Precursors of the Ilizarov technique. Injury 1993;2(Suppl):S25.

5. Lowenberg DW, Randall RL: The Ilizarov Method. In: Surgical Technolgy International II: International Developments in Surgery and Surgical Research. Ed. by Braverman MH and Tawes RL. San Francisco, Surgical Technology International, pp 459–462, 1993.

6. Draper ER, Wallace AL, Strachan RK, et al. The design and performance of an experimental external fixation device with load transducers. Med Eng Phys 1995;17:618–24.

7. Gardner TN, Hardy JR, Evans M, et al. The static and dynamic behaviour of tibial fractures due to unlocking external fixators. Clin Biomech (Bristol, Avon) 1996;11:425–30.

8. Gardner TN, Simpson H, Kenwright J. Rapid application fracture fixators—an evaluation of mechanical performance. Clin Biomech (Bristol, Avon) 2001;16:151–9.

9. Duda GN, Sollmann M, Sporrer S, et al. Interfragmentary motion in tibial osteotomies stabilized with ring fixators. Clin Orthop Relat Res 2002;396: 163–72.

10. Lowenberg DW, Nork S, Abruzzo FM. Correlation of shear to compression for progressive fracture obliquity. Clin Orthop Relat Res 2008;466(12): 2947–54.

11. Lenarz C, Bledsoe G, Watson JT. Circular external fixation frames with divergent half pins. Clin Orthop Relat Res 2008;466(12):2933–9.

12. Paley D, Herzenberg J. Applications of external fixation to foot and ankle reconstruction. Myerson M, editor In: Foot and ankle disorders, vol. 2 1984. P. 131-8;34:1135–88.

13. Foster PA, Barton SB, Jones SC, et al. The treatment of complex tibial shaft fractures by the Ilizarov method. J Bone Joint Surg Br 2012;94: 1678–83.

14. Hosny G, Fadel M. Ilizarov external fixator for open fractures of the tibial shaft. Int Orthop 2003;27(5): 303–6.

15. Tilkeridis K, Owen AJ, Royston SL, et al. The Ilizarov method for the treatment of segmental tibial fractures. Injury Extra 2009;40:228.

16. Keating J, Simpson A, Robinson C. The management of fractures with bone loss. J Bone Joint Surg Br 2005;87:142–50.

17. Ilizarov G, Ledyaev V. The replacement of long tubular bone defects by lengthening distraction osteotomy of one of the fragments: 1969. Clin Orthop 1992;(280):7–10.

18. Green S, Jackson J, Wall D, et al. Management of segmental defects by the Ilizarov intercalary bone transport method. Clin Orthop Relat Res 1992;(280):136–42.

19. Watson T, Coufal C. Treatment of complex lateral plateau fractures using Ilizarov techniques. Clin Orthop Relat Res 1998;353:97–106.

20. Raikin S, Froimson M. Combined limited internal fixation with circular frame external fixation of intra-articular tibial fractures. Orthopedics 1999; 22(11):1019–25.

21. Krupp A, Malkani A, Roberts C, et al. Treatment of bicondylar tibia plateau fractures using locked plating versus external fixation. Orthopedics 2009;32(8).

22. Dal Monte A, Donzelli O. Tibial lengthening according to Ilizarov in congenital hypoplasia of the leg. J Pediatr Orthop 1987;7:135.

23. Paley D, Catagni M, Argnani F, et al. Ilizarov treatment of tibial non-unions with bone loss. Clin Orthop 1989;241:146.

24. Green SA, Harris L, Wall DM, et al. The Rancho mounting technique for the Ilizarov method. A preliminary report. Clin Orthop Relat Res 1992;280: 104–16.

25. Calhoun JH, Li F, Ledbetter BR, et al. Biomechanics of the Ilizarov fixator for fracture fixation. Clin Orthop Relat Res 1992;280:15–22.

26. Roberts CS, Dodds JC, Perry K, et al. Hybrid external fixation of the proximal tibia: strategies to improve frame stability. J Orthop Trauma 2003;17: 415–20.

27. Augat P, Claes L, Hanselmann KF, et al. Increase of stability in external fracture fixation by hydroxyapatite-coated bone screws. J Appl Biomater 1995;6:99–104.

28. Young MJ, Barrack RL. Complications of internal fixation of tibial plateau fractures. Orthop Rev 1994;23:149 54.

29. Moore TM, Patzakis MJ, Harvey JP. Tibial plateau fractures: definition, demographics, treatment rationale, and long-term results of closed traction management or operative reduction. J Orthop Trauma 1987;1:97–119.

30. Mallik AR, Covall DJ, Whitelaw GP. Internal versus external fixation of bicondylar tibial plateau fractures. Orthop Rev 1992;21:1433–6.

31. Stamer DT, Schenk R, Staggers B, et al. Bicondylar tibial plateau fractures treated with a hybrid ring external fixator: a preliminary study. J Orthop Trauma 1994;8:455–61.

32. Buckle R, Blake R, Watson JT, et al. Treatment of the complex tibial plateau fractures with the Ilizarov external fixator. J Orthop Trauma 1993;7:167–8.

33. Watson JT. High-energy fractures of the tibial plateau. Orthop Clin North Am 1994;25:723–52.

34. Mikulak S, Gold S, Zinar D. Small wire fixation of high energy tibial plateau fractures. Clin Orthop Relat Res 1998;356:230–8.

35. Kumar A, Whittle P. Treatment of complex (Schatzker Type VI) fractures of the tibial plateau with circular wire external fixation: a retrospective case review. J Orthop Trauma 2000;14(5):339–44.

36. Canadian Orthopaedic Trauma Society. Open reduction and internal fixation compared with circular fixator application for bicondylar tibial plateau fractures. Results of a multicenter, prospective, randomized clinical trial. J Bone Joint Surg Am 2006;88(12):2613–23.

37. Katsenis D, Athanasiou V, Megas P, et al. Minimal internal fixation augmented by small wire transfixion frames for high-energy tibial plateau fractures. J Orthop Trauma 2005;19(4):241–8.

38. Marsh JL, Smith ST, Do TT. External fixation and limited internal fixation for complex fractures of the tibial plateau. J Bone Joint Surg Am 1995; 77(5):661–73.

39. Mahadeva D, Costa ML, Gaffey A. Open reduction and internal fixation versus hybrid fixation for bicondylar/severe tibial plateau fractures: a systematic review of the literature. Arch Orthop Trauma Surg 2008;128(10):1169–75.

40. Ramos T, Ekholm C, Eriksson B, et al. The Ilizarov external fixator—a useful alternative for the treatment of proximal tibia fractures. A prospective observational study of 30 consecutive patients. BMC Musculoskelet Disord 2013;14:11.

41. Tucker H, Kendra J, Kinnebrew T. Management of unstable open and closed tibial fractures using the Ilizarov method. Clin Orthop Relat Res 1992; 280:125–35.

42. El-Sayed M, Atef A. Management of simple (types A and B) closed tibial shaft fractures using percutaneous lag-screw fixation and Ilizarov external fixation in adults. Int Orthop 2012;36: 2133–8.

43. Sidharthan S, Sujith A, Rathod AK, et al. Management of high-energy tibial fractures using the Ilizarov apparatus. Internet J Orthop Surg 2005;2(2).

44. Wani N, Baba A, Kangoo K, et al. Role of early Ilizarov ring fixator in the definitive management of type II, IIIA, IIIB open tibial shaft fractures. Int Orthop 2011;35:915–23.

45. Oztürkmen Y, Karamehmetoğlu M, Karadeniz H, et al. Acute treatment of segmental tibial fractures with the Ilizarov method. Injury 2009;40:321–6.

46. Giotakis N, Panchani SK, Narayan B, et al. Segmental fractures of the tibia treated by circular external fixation. J Bone Joint Surg Br 2010;92-B: 687–92.

47. Sen C, Kocaoglu M, Eralp L, et al. Bifocal compression-distraction in the acute treatment of grade III open tibia fractures with bone and soft-tissue loss: a report of 24 cases. J Orthop Trauma 2004;18(3):150–7.

48. Hutson J, Dayicioglu D, Oeltjen J, et al. The treatment of Gustillo grade IIIB tibia fractures with application of antibiotic spacer, flap, sequential distraction osteogenesis. Ann Plast Surg 2010; 64(5):541–52.

49. Inan M, Halici M, Ayan I, et al. Treatment of type IIIA open fractures of tibial shaft with Ilizarov external fixator versus unreamed tibial nailing. Arch Orthop Trauma Surg 2007;127:617–23.

50. Teeny SM, Wiss DA. Open reduction and internal fixation of tibial plafond fractures: variables contributing to poor results and complications. Clin Orthop 1993;292:108–17.

51. Patterson M, Cole JD. Two staged delayed open reduction and internal fixation of severe pilon fractures. J Orthop Trauma 1999;13:85–91.

52. Lovisetti G, Agus MA, Pace F, et al. Management of distal tibial intra-articular fractures with circular external fixation. Strategies Trauma Limb Reconstr 2009;4:1–6.

53. Barbieri R, Schenk R, Koval K, et al. Hybrid external fixation in the treatment of tibial plafond fractures. Clin Orthop 1996;332:16–22.

54. Wyrsch B, McFerran MA, McAndrew M, et al. Operative treatment of fractures of the tibial plafond: a randomized, prospective study. J Bone Joint Surg Am 1996;78-A:1646–57.

55. Tornetta P 3rd, Weiner L, Bergman M, et al. Pilon fractures: treatment with combined internal and external fixation. J Orthop Trauma 1993;6:489–96.

56. McDonald MG, Burgess RC, Bolano LE, et al. Ilizarov treatment of pilon fractures. Clin Orthop 1996;325:232–8.

57. Bacon S, Smith WR, Morgan SJ, et al. A retrospective analysis of comminuted intra-articular fractures of the tibial plafond: open reduction and internal fixation versus external Ilizarov fixation. Injury 2008;39:196–202.

58. Kapoor SK, Kataria H, Patra SR, et al. Capsuloligamentotaxis and definitive fixation by an ankle-spanning Ilizarov fixator in high-energy pilon fractures. J Bone Joint Surg Br 2010;92:1100–6.

59. Kim HS, Jahng JS, Kim SS, et al. Treatment of tibial pilon fractures using ring fixators and arthroscopy. Clin Orthop 1997;334:244–50.

60. Kapukaya A, Subasi M, Arslan H, et al. Nonreducible, open tibial plafond fractures treated with a circular external fixator (is the current classification sufficient or identifying fractures in this area?). Injury 2005;36:1480–7.

61. Lowenberg DW, Sadeghi C, Brooks D, et al. Use of circular external fixation to maintain foot position during free tissue transfer to the foot and ankle. Microsurgery 2008;28(8):623–7.

62. Lowenberg DW, Parrett BM, Buntic RF, et al. Long term results and costs of muscle flap coverage with Ilizarov bone transport in lower limb salvage. J Orthop Trauma 2013;27(10):576–81.

Surgical Management of Isolated Greater Tuberosity Fractures of the Proximal Humerus

Daniel DeBottis, MD[a], Jack Anavian, MD[b],
Andrew Green, MD[a],*

KEYWORDS

- Proximal humerus fracture • Greater tuberosity fracture • Rotator cuff
- Open reduction and internal fixation • Glenohumeral dislocation • Arthroscopic internal fixation

KEY POINTS

- Because the greater tuberosity is the insertion site of the posterior superior rotator cuff, fractures can have a substantial impact on functional outcome.
- Although the greater tuberosity is commonly involved in proximal humerus fractures, isolated fractures are not and can be inadvertently trivialized.
- Thorough patient evaluation including adequate imaging is required to make an appropriate treatment decision.
- In most cases surgical management is considered when there is displacement of 5 mm or greater.
- Although reduction of displaced greater tuberosity fractures has traditionally been performed with open techniques, arthroscopic techniques are now available.
- The most reliable techniques of fixation of the greater tuberosity incorporate the rotator cuff tendon bone junction rather than direct bone-to-bone fixation.

INTRODUCTION

Although proximal humerus fractures account for approximately 5% of all fractures and many involve the tuberosities, isolated greater tuberosity fractures are less common and only account for about 2% of proximal humerus fractures.[1–3] The intimate association of the rotator cuff with the tuberosities has a substantial impact on the management and outcome of these injuries. In addition, age-related factors such as activity level and bone quality play a role in the treatment of greater tuberosity fractures. The appropriate management of these fractures is predicated on having a clear understanding of the relevant anatomy, fracture characteristics, associated injuries, and patient factors. This article focuses on current principles of surgical management of isolated greater tuberosity fractures.

ANATOMY

The greater tuberosity is an apophyseal structure of the proximal humerus. Ossification of the

Funding: None.
Conflicts of Interest: A. Green: Smith and Nephew, Arthrex, Synthes, unrestricted educational grant; Tornier, consulting and royalties. J. Anavian and D. DeBottis: none.
[a] Division of Shoulder and Elbow Surgery, Department of Orthopaedic Surgery, Warren Alpert Medical School of Brown University, Providence, RI, USA; [b] Department of Orthopaedic Surgery, Warren Alpert Medical School of Brown University, Providence, RI, USA
* Corresponding author. University Orthopedics, Inc, 2 Dudley Street, Suite 200, Providence, RI 02905.
E-mail address: agshoulder@aol.com

Orthop Clin N Am 45 (2014) 207–218
http://dx.doi.org/10.1016/j.ocl.2013.12.007
0030-5898/14/$ – see front matter © 2014 Elsevier Inc. All rights reserved.

greater tuberosity occurs during the second and third years of life. On average, the superior aspect of the greater tuberosity is 6 to 8 mm inferior to the most superior aspect of the articular surface of the humeral head[4] and is composed of 3 facets: superior, middle, and inferior.[5] Recent anatomic studies show that the rotator cuff tendon insertions on the greater tuberosity are more complex than earlier descriptions (**Fig. 1**).[5–7] An earlier anatomic study found that the supraspinatus tendon inserts on the superior facet and the superior half of the middle facet, whereas the infraspinatus tendon inserts on the entire middle facet, covering a portion of the supraspinatus tendon.[5] A more recent anatomic study by Mochizuki and colleagues[6] describes a different relationship in which the supraspinatus insertion is localized to the anteromedial aspect of the highest impression of the superior facet and the infraspinatus insertion is localized to the anterolateral aspect of the highest impression of the superior facet and all of the middle facet. The soft tissue attachments of the rotator cuff affect the direction and amount of displacement of the fractured greater tuberosity. The force vectors of the supraspinatus and upper aspect of the infraspinatus result in superior displacement, whereas the lower infraspinatus and teres minor cause posterior displacement. Understanding this anatomy helps to guide both the evaluation of injuries and the operative management of displaced fractures.

The vascularity of the greater tuberosity, as well as the humeral head articular segment, derives from an anastomosis of vessels from the posterior humeral circumflex vessels and the ascending branch of the anterior humeral circumflex artery (arcuate artery), and to a lesser degree by the rotator cuff tendons and joint capsule.[8,9] Hettrich and colleagues[9] performed a quantitative assessment of the blood supply to the humeral head and found that, overall, the posterior humeral circumflex artery contributes more to the blood supply (64%) than the anterior humeral circumflex artery (36%), including the area containing the greater tuberosity. Isolated fractures of the greater tuberosity have not proved to compromise blood flow to the humeral head.[10]

Proximal humerus fractures, including isolated greater tuberosity fractures, are commonly associated with neurologic injury. The axillary nerve, a branch of the posterior cord of the brachial plexus, passes inferior to the subscapularis muscle and through the quadrilateral space before dividing into anterior and posterior branches, which provide innervation to the deltoid and teres minor muscles respectively, as well as sensory innervation to the lateral aspect of the upper arm and shoulder. The axillary nerve is thus tethered anteriorly and posteriorly and subject to traction injury, especially with glenohumeral dislocation. The suprascapular nerve passing through suprascapular notch and around the scapular spine at the spinoglenoid notch provides innervation to the supraspinatus and infraspinatus muscles. Both of these important peripheral nerves, as well as the more proximal aspects of the brachial plexus, are susceptible to traumatic and iatrogenic injury.

FRACTURE CLASSIFICATION

Codman's[11] early observation that fracture patterns involving the proximal humerus fractures often occurred along the physeal scars of the proximal humerus formed the basis for Neer's[10] 4-part classification system. The humeral shaft,

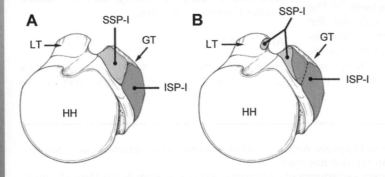

Fig. 1. The insertion of the rotator cuff tendons onto the greater tuberosity. (*A*) The generally accepted concept of the anatomy of the humeral insertions. The supraspinatus is shown to insert into the highest impression, and the infraspinatus into the middle impression of the greater tuberosity. (*B*) The findings of the present study. The insertion area of the infraspinatus occupies about half of the highest and all of the middle impression of the greater tuberosity. The insertion area of the supraspinatus is located at the anteromedial region of the highest impression and is sometimes located at the superior-most area on the lesser tuberosity. GT, greater tuberosity; HH, humeral head; ISP-I, insertion area of the infraspinatus; LT, lesser tuberosity; SSP-I, insertion area of the supraspinatus. (*From* Mochituki T, Sugaya H, Uomizu M, et al. Humeral insertion of the supraspinatus and infraspinatus. J Bone Joint Surg Am 2008;90:962–9; Figs. 6A and B; with permission.)

articular segment, and the greater and lesser tuberosities comprise the 4 parts of the proximal humerus. In the original description, 1 cm of displacement of 45° of angulation were the criteria that defined a part (**Fig. 2**).[10] This classification system emphasized the relationship between displacement and the rotator cuff, as well as displacement and the vascularity of the humeral head articular segment, and continues to be commonly used for the description of proximal humerus fractures. The AO/ASIF/OTA classification of proximal humerus fractures is based on the relationship between fracture fragments and the humeral head articular segment (**Fig. 3**).[12,13] Type A fractures are unifocal and involve the greater tuberosity or surgical neck. Similar to many other fracture classification systems, limited interobserver reliability has been shown.[14] Nevertheless, these classifications provide surgeons with useful information to define injuries and form the basis

for treatment, with displacement as the primary indication for considering surgical intervention.

In considering displacement of greater tuberosity fractures, both degree and direction are important. Healing with superior displacement can cause subacromial impingement, whereas posterior displacement can block external rotation motion.[15] More recent recommendations consider even a few millimeters of greater tuberosity displacement to be clinically relevant in some cases, and greater tuberosity displacement of more than 5 mm is an indication for operative treatment.[16] Park and colleagues[17] suggested that good results can be obtained with nonoperative treatment when the displacement is less than 5 mm. However, they also suggested that, if the displacement is more than 5 mm in young active patients, and more than 3 mm in athletes and heavy laborers with demand for overhead activity, the fracture should be repaired.[17]

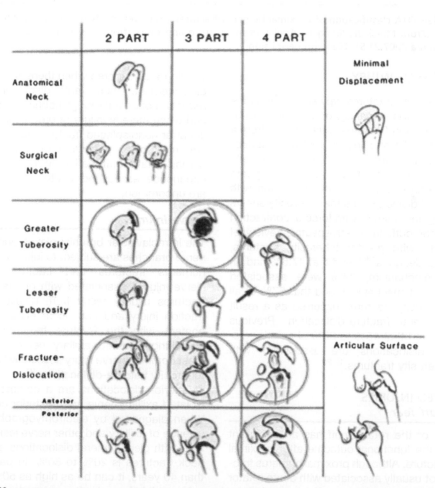

Fig. 2. Neer[10] classification of proximal humerus fractures. Fractures involving the greater tuberosity are highlighted. (*Adapted from* Neer CS II. Displaced proximal humerus fractures: part 1. Classification and evaluation. J Bone Joint Surg Am 1970;52:1077–89; with permission.)

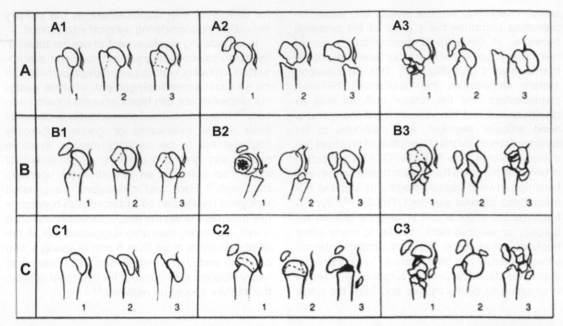

Fig. 3. AO/ASIF/OTA classification of proximal humerus fractures. Fractures involving the greater tuberosity are highlighted. (*From* Marsh JL, Slong TF, Agel J, et al. Fracture and dislocation classification compendium-2007. J Orthop Trauma 2007;21:S1–163; with permission.)

MECHANISM OF INJURY

Greater tuberosity fractures typically occur as the result of impaction, shearing, or avulsion mechanisms.[18] Impaction fractures usually occur from a direct fall onto the shoulder or with hyperabduction and compression of the greater tuberosity against the acromion. In contrast, shearing and avulsion fractures can occur in association with glenohumeral dislocation as the tuberosity shears across the glenoid rim or with forceful contraction of the rotator cuff. In a retrospective review of 103 patients with greater tuberosity fractures, Bahrs and colleagues[18] found that 47.6% had an impaction mechanism, 32% were associated with an indirect mechanism, and that 57% of all greater tuberosity fractures occurred as a result of glenohumeral fracture-dislocation. Previous studies showed that 15% to 30% of anterior glenohumeral dislocations are associated with greater tuberosity fractures.[19,20]

ASSOCIATED INJURIES
Rotator Cuff Tear

The status of the rotator cuff has an important impact on the functional outcome after proximal humerus facture. Although proximal humerus fractures are not usually associated with acute rotator cuff tears, preexisting rotator cuff tears and disorders are more common with advancing age. Associated acute rotator cuff tears can occur and

should be considered when there is marked initial displacement, persistent displacement after reduction of an anterior glenohumeral dislocation, and when there is failure of progression of recovery after nondisplaced fracture. Although also uncommon, older patients can have preexisting chronic rotator cuff tearing. In the senior author's experience associated acute rotator cuff tears are uncommon.

Nerve Injuries

The infraclavicular brachial plexus and peripheral nerve branches are subject to injury with proximal humerus fractures and fracture-dislocations. Nerve injuries associated with greater tuberosity fractures usually result from displacement and traction injury and can occur either from direct contact with the fracture fragments or from stretching. Isolated axillary nerve injury is the most common nerve injury associated with greater tuberosity fracture-dislocations.[21]

Anterior dislocations are a common cause of isolated axillary nerve and posterior cord lesions. When diagnosed by electromyography, the prevalence of axillary and other nerve lesions associated with glenohumeral dislocations and humeral neck fractures is 20% to 30%. In patients older than 40 years, it can be as high as 50%.[21–24]

Nerve injuries are often missed or overlooked in the acute setting because pain and immobilization can make examination difficult. Sensory deficit is especially difficult to assess and does not always accompany an axillary nerve lesion. However, recovery of nerve injuries associated with proximal humerus fractures is often incomplete. Alnot[25] reported that 80% of isolated axillary nerve lesions were neurapraxias that recovered in 4 to 6 months. Although persistent complete deltoid palsy is rare, a long delay before reinnervation lessens the likelihood of complete functional recovery.

Vascular Injuries

Although vascular injuries are rarely associated with proximal humeral fractures, the consequences of a missed injury are severe, thus highlighting the importance of early evaluation of the vascular status of the upper extremity. Axillary artery injury has been reported in approximately 5% of 4-part proximal humeral fractures.[21,26] Swelling and the collateral circulation may mask the extent of the vascular injury. Even in the presence of a complete axillary artery occlusion, the radial pulse may be palpable because of the extensive collateral circulation around the shoulder. The peripheral pulses, including the radial artery, should be palpated in addition to seeking other signs of vascular injury such as paresthesias, pallor or cyanosis, and an expanding hematoma. If a vascular injury is suspected, Doppler ultrasonography and arteriography should be performed and appropriate management emergently instituted in the case of significant arterial injury.

EVALUATION

The evaluation of a patient with an injured shoulder includes a history, physical examination, and diagnostic imaging. A complete history includes information about the patient's age, hand dominance, occupation, general health status, activity level, psychosocial status, details of the injury event, and any associated symptoms such as weakness or paresthesia suggesting neurologic involvement. The initial evaluation in the acute posttraumatic setting varies from a subacute presentation. In the acute setting, signs of neurovascular injury, glenohumeral dislocation, and other associated trauma should be sought. Axillary nerve motor function can be determined by assessing isometric muscle contraction of the deltoid muscle (**Fig. 4**). Axillary nerve sensory function can be assessed in the lateral deltoid region. However, this is not a reliable measure of axillary nerve function and may be misleading, because patients can have intact sensation in the axillary nerve distribution, but abnormal motor function.[15] External and

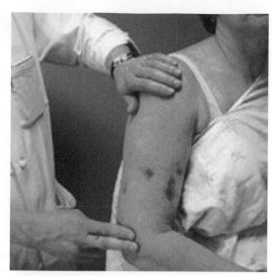

Fig. 4. Examination of deltoid muscle function in the acute postinjury phase.

internal rotation function can be grossly assessed with manual muscle testing but cannot be as accurately evaluated because these muscles cannot be directly palpated. Nevertheless, weakness, especially in older patients, should alert the examiner to the possibility of rotator cuff tear or displaced tuberosity fracture. Patients should undergo electrodiagnostic testing if nerve dysfunction has not resolved after 3 to 6 weeks.[15]

Radiographic evaluation should include a trauma series that consists of a true anteroposterior (AP) view of the glenohumeral joint, a scapular-Y view, and an axillary view (**Fig. 5**).[26] These views may be supplemented with additional internal and external rotation views when necessary. The visualization of the fracture, as well as the amount of displacement, varies depending on the specific projection viewed.[27] The size of the fracture fragments can vary from large, with or without comminution, to very small fragments seen in rotator cuff avulsion injuries. Fractures that are displaced posteriorly may overlap with the humeral head and be missed on an AP view and can be visualized posterior to the head on a scapular-Y view. In cases in which plain radiographs are unclear or further detailed imaging is needed, computed tomography imaging can be obtained.[28] Posterior displacement of the greater tuberosity can be assessed with axial imaging, whereas superior displacement can be evaluated with coronal imaging (**Fig. 6**).[15] Magnetic resonance imaging (MRI) is not routinely used in the diagnosis of displaced greater tuberosity fractures, because it does not often add information that alters treatment. However, it may

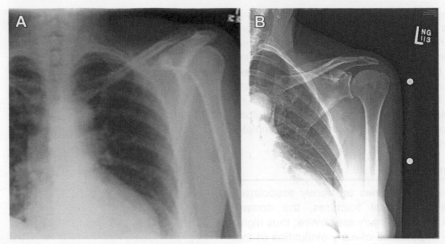

Fig. 5. (*A*) Initial plain radiographs failed to demonstrate the greater tuberosity fracture in this case. (*B*) Subsequent true anterior posterior radiograph demonstrated a non-displaced fracture.

be useful in making the diagnosis of occult, nondisplaced fractures[29] or associated rotator cuff tears (**Fig. 7**).

Inadequate radiographs may result in missed injuries such as an associated nondisplaced or minimally displaced fracture of the surgical or anatomic neck or lesser tuberosity. Closed reduction of an apparently isolated anterior greater tuberosity fracture-dislocation should be approached with caution because it can result in iatrogenic displacement of an initially nondisplaced surgical neck fracture.

TREATMENT
Nonoperative Treatment

Decision making in the management of isolated displaced greater tuberosity requires an understanding of the approach to management of nondisplaced or minimally displaced fractures. Nondisplaced fractures of the greater tuberosity are treated nonoperatively with good results expected.[10] A short period of immobilization is used to reduce pain and to prevent displacement of nonimpacted fractures and is followed by early initiation of passive range-of-motion exercises. Active elevation, abduction, and external rotation should be avoided early after injury. Most impacted greater tuberosity fractures are stable and range-of-motion exercises can begin within a week of injury.[26] McLaughlin[16] reported that displaced greater tuberosity fractures associated with anterior glenohumeral dislocation usually reduce with closed reduction. Reduced greater tuberosity fractures associated with fracture-dislocations are immobilized for a period of 2 weeks before motion exercises are started, to avoid redisplacement.[15]

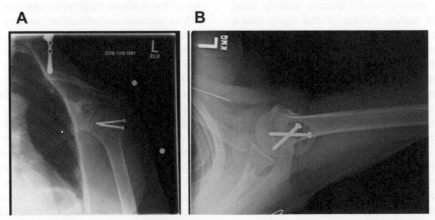

Fig. 6. True AP (*A*) and axillary lateral (*B*) radiographs of open reduction and internal fixation–isolated greater tuberosity fracture with screws.

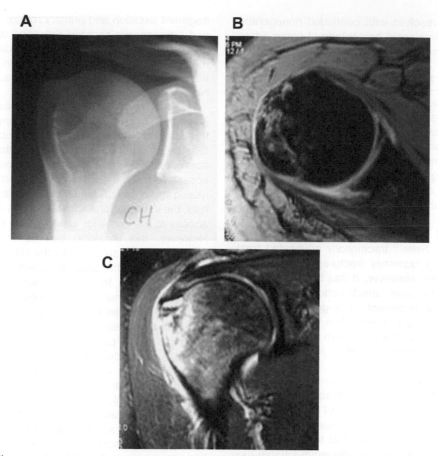

Fig. 7. (*A*) The true AP plain radiograph was unremarkable. However, the MRI showed an occult nondisplaced greater tuberosity. The coronal (*B*) and axial (*C*) images clearly show the fracture.

Serial radiographs are obtained to ensure that there is no displacement of the fracture fragment after motion is begun. Active range-of-motion exercises and progressive strengthening are begun at 6 weeks after the injury. More significant strengthening is delayed until the patient regains full passive motion.[15] The most common complication that occurs after nonoperative treatment of nondisplaced or minimally displaced isolated greater tuberosity fractures is shoulder stiffness.[30]

Platzer and colleagues[31] reported that 97% of patients with greater tuberosity fractures with less than 5 mm of displacement had good or excellent results after nonoperative treatment. In their series, female patients had significantly better results than male patients, and elderly patients had significantly worse results than younger patients.[31] Although not statistically significant, fracture displacement of more than 3 mm had slightly worse results than those with less displacement.[31] Rath and colleagues[32] studied a cohort of 69 patients who had nonoperative management of minimally displaced (<3 mm) greater tuberosity

fractures. At an average follow-up of 31 months (range, 26–41 months) the mean Constant score was 95 (range, 75–100) and the mean satisfaction score was 9.5 out of 10 (range, 7–10). They reported an average duration of pain and limited range of motion of 8 months.

However, not all patients have satisfactory results after nonoperative treatment of nondisplaced or minimally displaced fractures. In addition, historical reports show that nonoperative treatment of displaced greater tuberosity fractures result in poor outcomes.[16,33] Kim and Ha[30] retrospectively reviewed 23 patients who underwent arthroscopic treatment of chronic shoulder pain and reported that all patients had partial-thickness rotator cuff tears located on the tuberosity fracture area with varying depths. At an average of 29 months, 20 of the 23 patients had good or excellent results after either debridement or repair of the tear, with 19 returning to their previous levels of activity.[30]

In the senior authors' experience, posttraumatic stiffness is a common problem even with nondisplaced or minimally displaced fractures. In most cases this resolves with continued nonoperative treatment. In a small percentage of cases arthroscopic capsular release may be required.

Operative Treatment

Although there is agreement that surgery is indicated to treat displaced greater tuberosity fractures, questions remain about the amount of displacement that requires surgery and the ideal operative management **Box 1**. Surgical repair of displaced greater tuberosity fractures is recommended in order to prevent malunion, pain, stiffness, and alteration of rotator cuff function.[34]

There is some controversy surrounding the amount of displacement for which treatment is required. Neer[10] traditionally advocated treating proximal humerus fractures with 1 cm of displacement. However, it has been shown that patients can have unsatisfactory results after nonoperative treatment of a greater tuberosity with displacement of more than 5 mm.[16] Patients with fractures with even 3 mm of displacement may require surgery to fully restore overhead function.[17,30,35]

The goal of operative treatment is to restore the anatomic position of a displaced greater tuberosity, ensure that the integrity of the rotator cuff is preserved, and permit early range-of-motion exercises. The options for surgical treatment include closed reduction and percutaneous internal fixation, open reduction and internal fixation (ORIF),

---

> **Box 1**
> **Tactical steps for open reduction and internal fixation (ORIF) of displaced greater tuberosity fracture**
>
> Operative Steps for ORIF:
>
> 1. Patient positioning: allow for adequate surgical exposure and intraoperative imaging.
> 2. Surgical approach: deltopectoral or deltoid splitting.
> 3. Identify long head biceps tendon and rotator cuff interval as guides to the supraspinatus and greater tuberosity fragment. Assess greater tuberosity fragment for comminution.
> 4. Mobilize displaced greater tuberosity with traction sutures.
> 5. Prepare fracture bed on proximal humerus.
> 6. Reduce greater tuberosity fragment and achieve fixation.
> 7. Assess shoulder range of motion and fixation stability.

---

fragment excision and primary rotator cuff repair, and arthroscopic-assisted reduction and internal fixation.[36–38] Although excision of fracture fragments with rotator cuff repair has been described, this should not be performed because it may hinder rotator cuff healing.[15]

The surgical approach for open treatment of displaced greater tuberosity fractures can be through either the deltopectoral approach anteriorly or through a superior deltoid-splitting approach. The deltopectoral approach allows access to the greater tuberosity without compromising the origin of the deltoid muscle. Nevertheless, the deltopectoral approach does offer limited access to the posterior aspect of the rotator cuff. However, this limitation can be overcome by placing traction sutures into the rotator cuff progressively from the anterior aspect of the supraspinatus tendon to the posterior aspect of the infraspinatus tendon. In addition, a small skin hook can be used to reach behind the humerus and pull the greater tuberosity from a retracted posterior medial position.

The superior deltoid-splitting approach is performed through a skin incision placed in the Langer lines over the lateral aspect of the acromion. The deltoid muscle is split at the raphe between the anterior and middle deltoid and detached from the anterior aspect of the acromion. Splitting the muscle laterally is limited by the axillary nerve; approximately 5 cm in men and about 4.5 cm in women. Although this approach provides good access to the anterior and posterior aspects of the greater tuberosity, there are limitations reaching the surgical neck of the humerus for fixation if the fracture fragment is large. If more distal exposure is required the deltoid can be split further as long as the axillary nerve is identified and carefully dissected and protected.

Several fixation techniques are available, including screw fixation, heavy suture fixation, and suture anchor fixation. Although isolated screw fixation of these fractures has been described it is not feasible if the fragment is comminuted and should be used with caution because of the risk of further fracture or subsequent displacement.[37] If there is poor bone quality a screw can be placed distal to the fracture bed to serve as a post for a tension band construct. Heavy transosseous suture fixation is a preferable technique with sutures placed at the bone-tendon junction as opposed to through fragment. A figure-of-eight technique across the fracture site (**Fig. 8**) helps prevent over-reduction of the fragment. Intraoperative fluoroscopy can be used to assess fracture reduction, although direct visualization of the fracture reduction should be clear at the bony margins of the

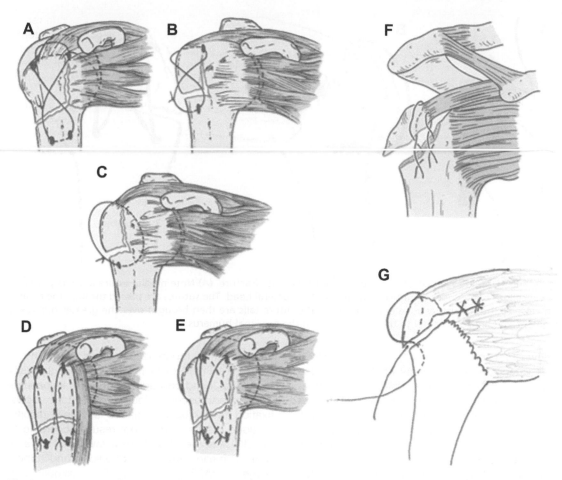

Fig. 8. Various suture fixation configurations for greater tuberosity fracture fixation. In (*F*) note that the suture crosses in the fracture and, when tied, prevents over-reduction of the greater tuberosity. Dashed lines, suture behind bone. (*From* Green A, Norris TR. Proximal humerus fractures and glenohumeral dislocations. Skeletal Trauma. 4th edition. In: Browner B, Jupiter J, Levine A, et al, editors. Philadelphia: WB Saunders; 2009; Figs. 44–55.)

greater tuberosity. In all cases extraneous dissection should be avoided to limit additional injury to the vascularity of the humeral articular segment. The anterior circumflex and the ascending branch are at risk with surgical dissection.

Closed reduction and percutaneous fixation is best reserved for cases with larger noncomminuted greater tuberosity fragments; typically in younger patients with good bone. Percutaneous fixation using pins and screws has been described, but this is also associated with failure of fixation.[36] Percutaneous instrumentation can be used to mobilize the greater tuberosity fragment into a reduced position.

Arthroscopic-assisted reduction can be combined with percutaneous or arthroscopic fixation. Suture-bridge fixation with medial and lateral anchors has been described for arthroscopic fixation and can also be used with open reduction.

The displaced fragment is reduced with 2 medial, transtendinous anchors and compressed to the fracture bed by fixing the sutures from the medial anchors with 2 lateral anchors placed beyond the fracture fragment (**Fig. 9**).[38] The construct strength of suture anchor fixation depends on bone quality and the type of anchor used.

Although several studies report on greater tuberosity fractures as part of larger series of proximal humerus fractures, there are few published data regarding the outcome of surgical management of isolated displaced greater tuberosity fractures. Jakob and colleagues[3] reported on a series of 930 operatively treated proximal humerus fractures, 17 of which were isolated greater tuberosity fractures, but did not report results. Paavolainen and colleagues[39] reported good results in 6 patients treated with screw fixation for an isolated greater tuberosity fracture. In a retrospective

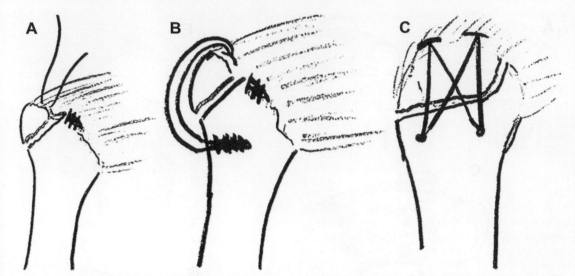

Fig. 9. Suture-bridge fixation of displaced greater tuberosity fracture. (*A*) Note medial suture anchors placed in the cancellous bone under the articular margin of the humeral head. The sutures are passed through the rotator cuff close to the tuberosity bone and tied. (*B, C*) The suture tails are then brought over the greater tuberosity fragment and anchored distal to the fracture bed in the proximal humerus.

review Chun and colleagues[40] reported results of 24 isolated greater tuberosity fractures included in a series of 141 2-part proximal humerus fractures. Ten of the 24 were treated with ORIF, 8 of which were fixed with screws. They reported follow-up data on only 11 of the 24 patients and they did not specify whether these were results of operative or nonoperative treatment.

Yin and colleagues[41] reported on 17 patients surgically treated for isolated displaced greater tuberosity fractures. Fifteen patients were treated with ORIF and 2 were treated arthroscopically. Radiographic union was achieved in 13 of the 15 patients with radiographic follow-up. At a follow-up of 5.2 years, the outcome was excellent in 11 (65%) patients, satisfactory in 5 (29%) patients, and unsatisfactory in 1 (6%) patient according to the Neer[10] criteria.

Flatow and colleagues[42] retrospectively reviewed 12 patients who underwent an anterosuperior deltoid-splitting approach with suture fixation for isolated greater tuberosity fractures. This approach, combined with rotation of the humerus, allowed adequate exposure of the retracted tuberosity.[42] All fractures healed, with 6 patients having excellent and 6 having good results at mean follow-up of 4.5 years.

Results from a recent biomechanical study by Lin and colleagues[43] comparing double-row and suture-bridge techniques to screw fixation suggest that using suture anchors provides stronger fixation than using screws. Suture anchor fixation was significantly better under cyclical load testing and ultimate load to failure. Several investigators

have recently reported outcomes after arthroscopic treatment of displaced greater tuberosity fractures. Ji and colleagues[44] treated 16 patients with an arthroscopic double-row suture anchor fixation technique and had 3 excellent results, 11 good results, and 2 poor results according to the UCLA score at a mean follow-up of 2 years with a mean American Shoulder and Elbow Surgeons (ASES) score of 88.1. Tsikouris and colleagues[45] reported outcomes in 12 athletes treated with arthroscopic reduction and fixation. Six of the 12 were professional athletes and all patients achieved radiographic union with all athletes returning to their preinjury activity levels.

MALUNION AND NONUNION

Malunion and nonunion of an isolated greater tuberosity fracture can result in substantial shoulder dysfunction. However, these are uncommon sequelae of injury. In contrast, many malunions and nonunions occur as a result of initial error in diagnosis either from inadequate imaging or underappreciation of the extent of injury. Depending on the size of the fragment, greater tuberosity nonunion causes variable rotator cuff weakness. The direction and degree of displacement of a malunited greater tuberosity determine the extent of weakness and limitation of motion.

Pain is the primary indication for treatment of an isolated greater tuberosity malunion or nonunion. Patients with painless limitation of function, except in cases of pseudoparalysis, do not usually present for further treatment. A malunited greater tuberosity can be corrected by either removing the prominent bone or by performing an osteotomy. The former technique is a reasonable option if the malunion is limited to the supraspinatus insertion. In this case the supraspinatus tendon can be elevated off the prominent greater tuberosity with or without a small bone fragment as if repairing a rotator cuff tear. Martinez and colleagues[16] described an arthroscopic technique in which the rotator cuff is detached, a tuberoplasty is performed, and the rotator cuff is repaired, and they reported good results in 8 patients. If there is preexisting rotator cuff tear, the prominent tuberosity is debrided and the rotator cuff tear is repaired. Osteotomy is preferred for larger fragments in order to take advantage of the better healing potential of bone to bone compared with tendon to bone. Greater tuberosity nonunions are repaired with similar techniques. However, if the tuberosity is displaced posteriorly it can be difficult to adequately mobilize the fragment, achieve stable fixation and healing, and at the same time avoid limitation of internal rotation. In cases with more severe dysfunction, especially in older patients, reverse total shoulder arthroplasty may be required to restore function.

SUMMARY

Among proximal humerus fractures, isolated greater tuberosity fractures are uncommon. For most patients, operative treatment with reduction and internal fixation is indicated for displacement of 5 mm. Individual patient factors dictate variation from this guideline for operative treatment.

REFERENCES

1. Kristinasen B, Barfod G, Bredesen J, et al. Epidemiology of proximal humerus fractures. Acta Orthop Scand 1987;58:75–7.
2. Court-Brown CM, Garg A, McQueen M. The epidemiology of proximal humerus fractures. Acta Orthop Scand 2001;72:365–71.
3. Jakob RP, Kristiansen T, Mayo K, et al. Classification and aspects of treatment of fractures of the proximal humerus. In: Bateman JE, Welsh RP, editors. Surgery of the shoulder. St Louis (MO): Mosby; 1984. p. 330–43.
4. Iannotti JP, Gabriel JP, Schneck SL, et al. The normal glenohumeral relationships: an anatomical study of one hundred and forty shoulders. J Bone Joint Surg Am 1992;74:491–500.
5. Minagawa H, Itoi E, Konno N, et al. Humeral attachment of the supraspinatus and infraspinatus: an anatomic study. Arthroscopy 1998;14:302–6.
6. Mochizuki T, Sugaya H, Uomizu M, et al. Humeral insertion of the supraspinatus and infraspinatus. J Bone Joint Surg Am 2008;90:962–9.
7. Curtis AS, Burbank KM, Tierney JJ, et al. The insertional footprint of the rotator cuff: an anatomic study. Arthroscopy 2006;22:603–9.
8. Brooks CH, Revell WJ, Heatley FW. Vascularity of the humeral head after proximal humeral fractures: an anatomical cadaver study. J Bone Joint Surg Br 1993;75:132–6.
9. Hettrich CM, Boraiah S, Dyke JP, et al. Quantitative assessment of the vascularity of the proximal part of the humerus. J Bone Joint Surg Am 2010;92:943–8.
10. Neer CS II. Displaced proximal humerus fractures: part 1. Classification and evaluation. J Bone Joint Surg Am 1970;52:1077–89.
11. Codman EA. Rupture of the supraspinatus tendon and other lesions in or about the subacromial bursa. Boston: Thomas Todd; 1934.
12. Muller ME, Allgower M, Schneider R, et al. Manual of internal fixation: techniques recommended by the AO-ASIF group. 3rd edition. New York: Springer-Verlag; 1995. p. 438–41.
13. Marsh JL, Slong TF, Agel J, et al. Fracture and dislocation classification compendium-2007. J Orthop Trauma 2007;21:S1–163.
14. Seibenrock KA, Gerber C. The reproducibility of classification of fractures of the proximal end of the humerus. J Bone Joint Surg Am 1993;75:1745–50.
15. Green A, Izzi J. Isolated fractures of the greater tuberosity of the proximal humerus. J Shoulder Elbow Surg 2003;12:641–9.
16. McLaughlin HL. Dislocation of the shoulder with tuberosity fracture. Surg Clin North Am 1963;43:1615–20.
17. Park TS, Choi IY, Kim YH, et al. A new suggestion for the treatment of minimally displaced fractures of the greater tuberosity of the proximal humerus. Bull Hosp Jt Dis 1997;56:171–6.
18. Bahrs C, Lingenfelter E, Fischer F, et al. Mechanism of injury and morphology of the greater tuberosity fracture. J Shoulder Elbow Surg 2006;15:140–7.
19. Rowe CR. Prognosis in dislocations of the shoulder. J Bone Joint Surg Am 1956;38:957–77.
20. Rowe CR, Sakellarides HT. Factors related to recurrences of anterior shoulder dislocations of the shoulder. Clin Orthop 1961;20:40–7.
21. Toolanen G, Hildingsson C, Hedlund T, et al. Early complications after anterior dislocation of the shoulder in patients over 40 years: an ultrasonographic and electromyographic study. Acta Orthop Scand 1993;64:549–52.
22. Bloom S, Dahlback LO. Nerve injuries in dislocations of the shoulder joint and fractures of the neck of the humerus: a clinical and electromyographic study. Acta Chir Scand 1970;136:461–6.

23. Pasila M, Jaroma H, Kiviluoto O, et al. Early complications of primary shoulder dislocations. Acta Orthop Scand 1978;49:260–3.

24. Stableforth PG. Four-part fractures of the neck of the humerus. J Bone Joint Surg Br 1984;66:104–8.

25. Alnot JY. Traumatic brachial plexus palsy in the adult: retro and infraclavicular lesions. Clin Orthop Relat Res 1988;237:9–16.

26. Green A, Norris TR. Proximal humerus fractures and glenohumeral dislocations. In: Browner B, Jupiter J, Levine A, et al, editors. Skeletal trauma. 4th edition. Philadelphia: Saunders; 2009. p. 1623–753.

27. Parsons BO, Klepps SJ, Miller S, et al. Reliability and reproducibility of radiographs of greater tuberosity fractures: a cadaveric study. J Bone Joint Surg Am 2005;87:58–65.

28. Burnstein J, Adler IM, Blank JE, et al. Evaluation of the Neer system of classification of proximal humerus fractures with computerized tomographic scans and plain radiographs. J Bone Joint Surg Am 1996;78:1371–5.

29. Reinus WR, Hatem SF. Fractures of the greater tuberosity presenting as rotator cuff abnormality: magnetic resonance demonstration. J Trauma 1998;44: 670–5.

30. Kim SH, Ha KI. Arthroscopic treatment of symptomatic shoulders with minimally displaced greater tuberosity fracture. Arthroscopy 2000;16: 695–700.

31. Platzer P, Kutscha-Lissberg F, Lehr S, et al. The influence of displacement on shoulder function in patients with minimally displaced fractures of the greater tuberosity. Injury 2005;36:1185–9.

32. Rath E, Alkrinawi N, Levy O, et al. Minimally displaced fractures of the greater tuberosity: outcome of non-operative treatment. J Shoulder Elbow Surg 2013;22(10):e8–11.

33. Santee HE. Fractures about the upper end of the humerus. Ann Surg 1924;80:103–14.

34. Bono CM, Renard R, Levine RG. Effect of displacement of fractures of the greater tuberosity on the mechanics of the shoulder. J Bone Joint Surg Br 2001;83:1056–62.

35. Platzer P, Thalhammer F, Oberleitner G, et al. Displaced fractures of the greater tuberosity: a comparison of operative and nonoperative treatment. J Trauma 2008;65:843–8.

36. Williams GR, Wong KL. Two-part and three-part fractures: open reduction and internal fixation versus closed reduction and percutaneous pinning. Orthop Clin North Am 2000;31:1–21.

37. Green A, Norris T. Complications of non-operative management and internal fixation of proximal humerus fractures. In: Flatow E, Ulrich C, editors. Musculoskeletal trauma series–humerus. Oxford (United Kingdom): Butterworth-Heinemann; 1996. p. 106–20.

38. Song HS, Williams GR Jr. Arthroscopic reduction and fixation with suture-bridge technique for displaced or comminuted greater tuberosity fractures. Arthroscopy 2008;24:956–60.

39. Paavolainen P, Bjorkenheim JM, Slatis P, et al. Operative treatment of severe proximal humeral fracture. Acta Orthop Scand 1983;54:374–9.

40. Chun JM, Groh GI, Rockwood CA Jr. Two-part fractures of the proximal humerus. J Shoulder Elbow Surg 1994;3:273–87.

41. Yin B, Moen TC, Thompson SA, et al. Operative treatment of isolated greater tuberosity fractures: retrospective review of clinical and functional outcomes. Orthopedics 2012;35:e807–14.

42. Flatow EL, Cuomo F, Maday MG, et al. Open reduction and internal fixation of two-part displaced fractures of the greater tuberosity of the proximal part of the humerus. J Bone Joint Surg Am 1991;73: 1213–8.

43. Lin CL, Hong CK, Jou IM, et al. Suture anchor versus screw fixation for greater tuberosity fractures of the humerus–a biomechanical study. J Orthop Res 2012;30:423–8.

44. Ji JH, Shafi M, Song IS, et al. Arthroscopic fixation technique for comminuted, displaced greater tuberosity fracture. Arthroscopy 2010;26:600–9.

45. Tsikouris G, Intzirtis P, Zampiakis E, et al. Arthoscopic reduction and fixation of fractures of the greater humeral tuberosity in athletes: a case series. Br J Sports Med 2013;47:v-e3.

46. Martinez AA, Calvo A, Domingo J, et al. Arthroscopic treatment for malunions of the proximal humeral greater tuberosity. Int Orthop 2010;34: 1207–11.

Upper Extremity

Preface
Upper Extremity

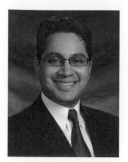

Asif M. Ilyas, MD
Editor

In this issue of the *Orthopedic Clinics of North America*, we present several interesting articles in the Upper Extremity section reviewing a number of upper extremity conditions.

Gutowski and I present a detailed review of the evaluation and medical management of osteoporosis, a condition that continues to grow in prevalence. The upper extremity is a common site to encounter osteoporosis-related fragility fractures and surgeons treating these injuries would benefit from an understanding of the symptoms, evaluation, and medical treatment options.

Abzug and Kozin provide a comprehensive review of brachial plexus birth palsies. Despite being well recognized, brachial plexus birth palsies continue to be relatively common, potentially resulting in permanent deficits in upper extremity function. The authors review the mechanism of injury, risk factors, anatomy, diagnosis, classification, and both surgical and nonsurgical treatment options.

Frank and colleagues present a detailed review of acromioplasty and discuss its role in the management of rotator cuff injuries. As the indication for performing an acromioplasty during rotator cuff surgery has recently been brought into question, the authors present the best recent evidence related to its utilization.

Asif M. Ilyas, MD
Rothman Institute
Thomas Jefferson University
925 Chestnut Street
Philadelphia, PA 19107, USA

E-mail address:
asif.ilyas@rothmaninstitute.com

http://dx.doi.org/10.1016/j.ocl.2014.01.001
0030-5898/14/$ – see front matter

orthopedic.theclinics.com

The Role of Acromioplasty for Rotator Cuff Problems

Jonathan M. Frank, MD[a],*, Jaskarndip Chahal, MD, FRCSC[b],
Rachel M. Frank, MD[a], Brian J. Cole, MD, MBA[c],
Nikhil N. Verma, MD[c], Anthony A. Romeo, MD[c]

KEYWORDS

- Acromioplasty • Subacromial decompression • Impingement syndrome • Rotator cuff repair

KEY POINTS

- Acromioplasty is a well-described technique used for a variety of rotator cuff pathologies, with a rapid rise in its use over the past several years.
- There are 2 competing theories regarding rotator cuff pathology—intrinsic and extrinsic—that either support or limit the potential benefits of acromioplasty.
- Acromioplasty may be an effective treatment option for subacromial impingement refractory to conservative therapy.
- The utility of acromioplasty at the time of rotator cuff repair has come into question, with new studies showing no significant benefit.
- Further studies with long-term follow-up are required to determine the efficacy of acromioplasty for impingement syndrome and during rotator cuff repair.

INTRODUCTION

In 1972, Neer first described acromioplasty and reported on its utility in treating chronic impingement syndrome.[1] He postulated acromial morphology as the initiating factor leading to dysfunction of the rotator cuff and eventual tearing.[1,2] This tenet is the basis for the extrinsic theory of rotator cuff degeneration and has had a profound impact on surgical practice, with several investigators advocating for concomitant acromioplasty during surgical repair of rotator cuff tears.[3–6] According to Neer's original description of the acromioplasty procedure, the anterior edge and undersurface of the anterior acromion is removed as well as the coracoacromial ligament. Since then, various modifications have been proposed. For example, in 1987, Ellman[7] described an arthroscopic technique to accomplish coracoacromial ligament release, resection of the anterior acromion undersurface, and bursal débridement, which he termed, *arthroscopic subacromial decompression (SAD).* McCallister and colleagues[8] as well as Matsen and Lippitt[9] described a "smooth and move," which involves an extensive bursectomy and smoothing of the undersurface of the acromion without altering acromial morphology. A potential complication of acromioplasty is postoperative avulsion of the deltoid origin due to its weakening by the procedure.[1,10] In order to avoid this, the smoothing procedure does not involve resection or release of the coracoacromial ligament.

The authors report no actual or potential conflict of interest in relation to this article.
[a] Department of Orthopaedic Surgery, Rush University Medical Center, 1653 West Congress Parkway, Chicago, IL 60612, USA; [b] Sports Medicine Program, Division of Orthopaedic Surgery, Department of Surgery, Women's College Hospital, University of Toronto, 55 Queen Street East, Suite 800, Toronto, ON, M5C 1R6, Canada; [c] Division of Sports Medicine, Midwest Orthopaedics at Rush, 1611 West Harrison Street, Suite 400, Chicago, IL 60612, USA
* Corresponding author.
E-mail address: jon.m.frank@gmail.com

In contrast to the extrinsic theory, the intrinsic theory of rotator cuff pathology proposes that abnormalities of the rotator cuff occur secondary to intratendinous degeneration or tendinosis, which in turn results when eccentric tensile overload occurs at a rate greater than the ability of the cuff to repair itself.[3] According to this perspective, acromioplasty as a form of treatment fails to address the aforementioned primary problem of intratendinous degeneration.

Recent epidemiologic studies have clearly demonstrated a rapid rise in the number of acromioplasty procedures performed in the United States on an annual basis. Vitale and colleagues[11] reviewed the records from the New York Statewide Planning and Research Cooperative System (SPARCS) ambulatory surgery database from 1996 to 2006 and the American Board of Orthopaedic Surgery (ABOS) database from 1999 to 2008 to identify patients who had an acromioplasty. The investigators found a 254.4% increase in the SPARCS group versus 142.3% in the ABOS group for the number of acromioplasties over their respective time-periods. Yu and colleagues[12] reviewed the records of 246 patients identified from the Rochester Epidemiology Project, cataloging medical records of residents in Olmsted County, Minnesota, who had an isolated acromioplasty performed between 1980 and 2005. They found a 575.8% increase over this time period, further demonstrating the widespread popularity of this procedure. Although there are many possible explanations for the observed increase in the annual number of acromioplasties, there is a need to evaluate whether this observed rise is associated with sound clinical indications supported by high-level clinical evidence.

At the present time, the 2 most common indications for performing an acromioplasty are subacromial impingement refractory to nonoperative care and during arthroscopic or open rotator cuff repair. The purpose of this article is to summarize and review the current evidence regarding the efficacy of acromioplasty both for subacromial impingement syndrome (SAIS) and during arthroscopic repair of rotator cuff tears.

ACROMIOPLASTY FOR MANAGEMENT OF SUBACROMIAL IMPINGEMENT SYNDROME

Rotator cuff disease with subacromial impingement has been described in 3 stages: stage 1, acute inflammation and either tendonitis or bursitis; stage 2, chronic inflammation with or without degeneration; and stage 3, full rupture of the cuff.[13] Subacromial impingement occurs when the normal sliding mechanism, while lifting the arm, is disrupted by compression of the soft tissues between the coracoacromial arch and the greater humeral tuberosity.[14] Patients complain of pain over the anterolateral shoulder, radiating down the lateral humerus.[15] They also report pain when laying on the affected extremity, oftentimes awakening them at night. Activities of daily living, such as combing hair or reaching for an item in a cupboard, are painful. Neer and Hawkins tests are 2 provocative examination maneuvers that are highly sensitive but not specific to subacromial impingement. Combined, they have a negative predictive value of 90%.[16]

Initial conservative management for SAIS includes nonsteroidal antiinflammatory drugs, physical therapy (PT), and corticosteroid injections. Few studies have looked at each of these modalities separately to determine their respective efficacy. Desmeules and colleagues[17] performed a systematic review evaluating the effectiveness of PT in treating impingement syndrome. In their review of 7 studies, they found that evidence did not support PT as an effective modality. More recently, however, Hanratty and colleagues[18] performed a systematic review and meta-analysis that included 16 studies (4 high quality, 7 medium quality, and 5 low quality) regarding PT in patients with subacromial impingement. They concluded that there was strong support for exercise in decreasing pain and improving function at short-term follow-up. There was also moderate evidence that exercise results in short-term improvement in mental well-being and a long-term improvement in function.

The current belief is that SAD is the gold standard surgical treatment. Several studies, however, have brought this into question. Brox and colleagues[19,20] (level 4, grade B-C) compared the outcomes of patients with stage 2 impingement, dividing them into 3 groups—PT, SAD, and placebo. They found that PT and SAD were each better than placebo but found no difference between the PT and SAD groups at 6 and at 30 months. Haahr and colleagues[21] (level 4, grade C) performed a randomized control study with 1-year follow-up comparing exercise to SAD. They found no statistically significant difference in the mean change in Constant scores between groups at 3, 6, and 12 months or in the Project on Research and Intervention in Monotonous Work (PRIM) scores (aggregated pain and dysfunction score) at 12 months. Rahme and colleagues[22] (level 4, grade C) compared open SAD to a physiotherapy regimen. At 6 and 12 months, there was no statistically significant difference between groups. Thus, these 3 studies, albeit of low quality, found no difference between SAD and conservative therapy.[23]

More recently, Ketola and colleagues[24] (level 1) performed a 2-year randomized controlled trial (RCT) comparing a supervised exercise program with arthroscopic acromioplasty followed by a supervised exercise program, with the main outcome measure self-reported pain on a visual analog scale (VAS). Although both groups showed an improvement, there was no statistically significant difference in the degree of improvement between groups on the VAS nor in secondary outcome measures of disability, pain at night, shoulder disability questionnaire score, number of painful days, and proportion of pain-free patients. The investigators note, however, that it seemed the operative group recovered faster in all parameters when assessed from the initiation of the treatment. At this time, the evidence does not seem to support acromioplasty over therapy and exercise and places in question its status as the gold standard of treatment of SAIS.

A study by Magaji and colleagues[25] (level 3) investigated the efficacy of SAD in patients with SAIS refractory to conservative therapy for 6 months. They found that patients with all of the following 4 criteria were excellent candidates for SAD: pain in the shoulder with overhead activity or in the midarc of abduction; a repeatedly positive Hawkins test; temporary pain relief (minimum 2 weeks) after subacromial steroid injection; and radiologic evidence of impingement with sclerosis, cysts, or osteophytes at the greater tuberosity and acromion. Perhaps the key to obtaining successful outcomes with surgical intervention lies in using strict criteria for identifying appropriate patients for SAD—that is, patients who have failed a prolonged nonoperative regimen for a minimum of 6 months, including supervised physical therapy, injections, and activity modification.

ACROMIOPLASTY DURING ARTHROSCOPIC ROTATOR CUFF REPAIR

There several pros and cons associated with performing an acromioplasty during arthroscopic rotator cuff repair. Advantages of performing an acriomioplasty include improved arthroscopic visualization and ability to control bleeding in the subacromial space as well as an increase in the local concentrations of growth and angiogenic factors, potentially improving the healing environment.[26,27] Possible disadvantages include weakening of the deltoid origin, a risk of anterosuperior instability in the presence of a failed rotator cuff or irreparable tear,[28,29] and adhesions between the raw exposed bone on the undersurface

of the acromion and the underlying tendon can form, which in turn can limit smoothness, motion, comfort, and range of motion.[30–32]

Traditionally, acromioplasty has routinely been performed as part of a rotator cuff repair. This stems from Neer's extrinsic theory of subacromial impingement. In the late 1990s, however, the intrinsic theory began to take hold, postulating that overuse and injury to the rotator cuff initiates as cascade that leads to narrowing of the subacromial space and a secondary impingement.[3] A recent systematic review by Seitz and Michener,[33] looking at ultrasonographic measurement of the subacromial space in patients with rotator cuff tears, seems to support this theory. Using 5 studies, they found that individuals with full-thickness cuff tears had a statistically significant decrease in the acromiohumeral distance compared with normal patients and even those with SAIS. This suggests that the pathoanatomy of cuff disease results in a secondary impingement and that perhaps addressing the cuff disease alone may secondarily ameliorate the impingement effect.

Testing whether a cuff repair without acromioplasty would still show significant improvement, McCallister and colleagues[8] (level 4) performed 96 consecutive full-thickness rotator cuff repairs without acromioplasty as part of a prospective cohort study. They looked at self-assessment of shoulder function with the Simple Shoulder Test and general health status with the Short Form-36 questionnaire. Of the 61 patients who participated in the study with a minimum 2-year follow-up, statistically significant improvement in shoulder comfort and function was noted, thereby bringing into question whether acromioplasty did improve outcomes.

Several high-level studies have attempted to investigate whether acromioplasty is a necessary part of a rotator cuff repair. Gartsman and O'connor[34] (level 1) performed a prospective RCT comparing rotator cuff repair with acromioplasty versus without with a minimum of 1-year follow-up. They found no statistical difference in the American Shoulder and Elbow Surgeons (ASES) shoulder scores between groups, with the conclusion that acromioplasty does not affect functional outcome after cuff repair.

Milano and colleagues[35] (level 1) evaluated the role of SAD in rotator cuff repair in a prospective RCT of 80 patients divided equally between groups with a minimum 2-year follow-up. They found no difference either in the Constant score, which was normalized for age and gender, or in the Disabilities of the Arm, Shoulder and Hand (DASH) and Work-DASH scores. Thus, they also concluded that SAD did not alter outcomes of rotator cuff repair.

MacDonald and colleagues[36] (level 1) compared functional and quality-of-life indices and rates of revision surgery in arthroscopic rotator cuff repair with and without acromioplasty in a prospective RCT. They used the Western Ontario Rotator Cuff Index (WORC) score as the primary outcome and the ASES score as a secondary outcome. Also reviewed were the numbers of revision surgeries required. No difference was found in the WORC or ASES scores at any time point. They did find a strong trend, however, in the number of patients who required reoperation in the nonacromioplasty group ($P = .05$).

Combining these 3 prospective RCTs as well as an unpublished RCT,[37] Chahal and colleagues[38] conducted a level 1 systematic review and meta-analysis evaluating the role of SAD in full-thickness rotator cuff repairs in 373 patients. A quantitative synthesis demonstrated no significant difference in functional outcomes (Constant and ASES scores) or the rate of reoperation in the first 2 years after surgery.

Most recently, Shin and colleagues[39] (level 2) performed a randomized comparative study investigating the role of acromioplasty at the time of arthroscopic rotator cuff repair in patients with small- to medium-sized tears. They found no significant difference in range of motion or VAS, ASES, Constant, and University of California, Los Angeles, scores between groups. There was also no statistically significant difference in the rate of rotator cuff repair failure as assessed by postoperative MRI.

At this time, the American Academy of Orthopaedic Surgeons clinical practice guidelines for the treatment of rotator cuff tears do not recommend routine acromioplasty during rotator cuff repair.[40] Based on the best available evidence today, the authors fully endorse that there are no benefits in measured outcomes at up to 2 years after surgery; however, the long-term effects of performing or not performing an acromioplasty at the time of rotator cuff repair are not known. It may be possible that certain groups do benefit from acromioplasty (eg, acquired type 3, lateral downslope). Larger well-designed RCTs will allow investigators to perform the appropriate subgroup analyses to address these issues.

SUMMARY

Long-term follow-up with stratification for acromion type and workers' compensation status is required to determine the efficacy of acromioplasty for impingement syndrome and during rotator cuff repair. Furthermore, in the setting of SAIS, there are no studies comparing SAD with combined injection (cortisone and platelet-rich plasma) and PT regimens. For both of the aforementioned clinical indications for acromioplasty, outcome measures of interest should be uniformly reported and include a disease-specific quality-of-life measure (WORC), a generic patient-reported outcome measure (DASH, ASES, or Constant score), objective deltoid strength measurement, and postoperative imaging to evaluate acromial morphology, rotator cuff healing, and the presence of anterosuperior escape in the setting of failed or new rotator cuff tears.

REFERENCE

1. Neer CS. Anterior acromioplasty for the chronic impingement syndrome in the shoulder: a preliminary report. J Bone Joint Surg Am 2006;54(1):41–50.
2. Bigliani LU, Ticker JB, Flatow EL, et al. The relationship of acromial architecture to rotator cuff disease. Clin Sports Med 1991;10(4):823–38.
3. Budoff JE, Nirschl RP, Guidi EJ. Current concepts review - débridement of partial-thickness tears of the rotator cuff without acromioplasty. Long-term follow-up and review of the literature. J Bone Joint Surg Am 1998;80(5):733–48.
4. Hawkins RJ, Misamore GW, Hobeika PE. Surgery for full-thickness rotator-cuff tears. J Bone Joint Surg Am 1985;67(9):1349–55.
5. Blevins FT, Warren RF, Cavo C, et al. Arthroscopic assisted rotator cuff repair: results using a mini-open deltoid splitting approach. Arthroscopy 1996; 12(1):50–9.
6. Romeo AA, Hang DW, Bach BR, et al. Repair of full thickness rotator cuff tears. Gender, age, and other factors affecting outcome. Clin Orthop Relat Res 1999;367:243–55.
7. Ellman H. Arthroscopic subacromial decompression: analysis of one- to three-year results. Arthroscopy 1987;3(3):173–81.
8. McCallister WV, Parsons IM, Titelman RM, et al. Open rotator cuff repair without acromioplasty. J Bone Joint Surg Am 2005;87(6):1278–83. http://dx.doi.org/10.2106/JBJS.D.02432.
9. Matsen FA III, Lippitt SB. Procedure: smooth and move—cuff intact. In: Matsen FA III, Lippitt SB, editors. Shoulder surgery: principles and procedures. Philadelphia: Saunders; 2008. p. 328–46.
10. Sher JS, Iannotti JP, Warner JJ, et al. Surgical treatment of postoperative deltoid origin disruption. Clin Orthop Relat Res 1997;343:93–8.
11. Vitale MA, Arons RR, Hurwitz S, et al. The Rising Incidence of Acromioplasty. J Bone Joint Surg Am 2010;92(9):1842–50. http://dx.doi.org/10.2106/JBJS.I.01003.

12. Yu E, Cil A, Harmsen WS, et al. Arthroscopy and the dramatic increase in frequency of anterior acromioplasty from 1980 to 2005: an epidemiologic study. Arthroscopy 2010;26(Suppl 9):S142. http://dx.doi.org/10.1016/j.arthro.2010.02.029.

13. Frieman BG, Albert TJ, Fenlin JM. Rotator cuff disease: a review of diagnosis, pathophysiology, and current trends in treatment. Arch Phys Med Rehabil 1994;75(5):604–9.

14. Huisstede BM, Miedema HS, Verhagen AP, et al. Multidisciplinary consensus on the terminology and classification of complaints of the arm, neck and/or shoulder. Occup Environ Med 2007;64:313–9. http://dx.doi.org/10.1136/oem.2005.023861.

15. Koester MC, George MS, Kuhn JE. Shoulder impingement syndrome. Am J Med 2005;118(5):452–5. http://dx.doi.org/10.1016/j.amjmed.2005.01.040.

16. MacDonald PB, Clark P, Sutherland K. An analysis of the diagnostic accuracy of the Hawkins and Neer subacromial impingement signs. J Shoulder Elbow Surg 2000;9(4):299–301. http://dx.doi.org/10.1067/mse.2000.106918.

17. Desmeules F, Côté CH, Frémont P. Therapeutic exercise and orthopedic manual therapy for impingement syndrome: a systematic review. Clin J Sport Med 2003;13(3):176–82.

18. Hanratty CE, McVeigh JG, Kerr DP, et al. The Effectiveness of physiotherapy exercises in subacromial impingement syndrome: a systematic review and meta-analysis. Semin Arthritis Rheum 2012;42(3):297–316. http://dx.doi.org/10.1016/j.semarthrit.2012.03.015.

19. Brox JI, Staff PH, Ljunggren AE, et al. Arthroscopic surgery compared with supervised exercises in patients with rotator cuff disease (stage II impingement syndrome). BMJ 1993;307(6909):899–903.

20. Brox JI, Gjengedal E, Uppheim G, et al. Arthroscopic surgery versus supervised exercises in patients with rotator cuff disease (stage II impingement syndrome): a prospective, randomized, controlled study in 125 patients with a 2 1/2-year follow-up. J Shoulder Elbow Surg 1999;8(2):102–11.

21. Haahr JP, Østergaard S, Dalsgaard J, et al. Exercises versus arthroscopic decompression in patients with subacromial impingement: a randomised, controlled study in 90 cases with a one year follow up. Ann Rheum Dis 2005;64(5):760–4.

22. Rahme H, Solem-Bertoft E, Westerberg CE, et al. The subacromial impingement syndrome. A study of results of treatment with special emphasis on predictive factors and pain-generating mechanisms. Scand J Rehabil Med 1998;30(4):253–62.

23. Dorrestijin O, Stevens M, Winters JC, et al. Conservative or surgical treatment for subacromial impingement syndrome? A systematic review. J Shoulder Elbow Surg 2009;18(4):652–60. http://dx.doi.org/10.1016/j.jse.2009.01.010.

24. Ketola S, Lehtinen J, Arnala I, et al. Does arthroscopic acromioplasty provide any additional value in the treatment of shoulder impingement syndrome?: a two-year randomised controlled trial. J Bone Joint Surg Br 2009;91(10):1326–34. http://dx.doi.org/10.1302/0301-620X.91B10.22094.

25. Magaji SA, Singh HP, Pandey RK. Arthroscopic subacromial decompression is effective in selected patients with shoulder impingement syndrome. J Bone Joint Surg Br 2012;94(8):1086–9. http://dx.doi.org/10.1302/0301-620X.94B8.29001.

26. Galliera E, Randelli P, Dogliotti G, et al. Matrix metalloproteases MMP-2 and MMP-9: are they early biomarkers of bone remodelling and healing after arthroscopic acromioplasty? Injury 2010;41(11):1204–7. http://dx.doi.org/10.1016/j.injury.2010.09.024.

27. Randelli P, Margheritini F, Cabitza P, et al. Release of growth factors after arthroscopic acromioplasty. Knee Surg Sports Traumatol Arthrosc 2008;17(1):98–101. http://dx.doi.org/10.1007/s00167-008-0653-4.

28. Fagelman M, Sartori M, Freedman KB, et al. Biomechanics of coracoacromial arch modification. J Shoulder Elbow Surg 2007;16(1):101–6. http://dx.doi.org/10.1016/j.jse.2006.01.010.

29. Lee TQ, Black AD, Tibone JE, et al. Release of the coracoacromial ligament can lead to glenohumeral laxity: a biomechanical study. J Shoulder Elbow Surg 2001;10(1):68–72. http://dx.doi.org/10.1067/mse.2001.111138.

30. Liu SH, Panossian V, al-Shaikh R, et al. Morphology and matrix composition during early tendon to bone healing. Clin Orthop Relat Res 1997;339:253–60.

31. Goldberg BA, Nowinski RJ, Matsen FA. Outcome of nonoperative management of full-thickness rotator cuff tears. Clin Orthop Relat Res 2001;382:99–107.

32. Romeo AA, Loutzenheiser T, Rhee YG, et al. The humeroscapular motion interface. Clin Orthop Relat Res 1998;350:120–7.

33. Seitz AL, Michener LA. Ultrasonographic measures of subacromial space in patients with rotator cuff disease: a systematic review. J Clin Ultrasound 2011;39(3):146–54. http://dx.doi.org/10.1002/jcu.20783.

34. Gartsman GM, O'connor DP. Arthroscopic rotator cuff repair with and without arthroscopic subacromial decompression: a prospective, randomized study of one-year outcomes. J Shoulder Elbow Surg 2004;13(4):424–6. http://dx.doi.org/10.1016/S1058274604000527.

35. Milano G, Grasso A, Salvatore M, et al. Arthroscopic rotator cuff repair with and without subacromial decompression: a prospective randomized study. Arthroscopy 2007;23(1):81–8. http://dx.doi.org/10.1016/j.arthro.2006.10.011.

36. MacDonald P, McRae S, Leiter J, et al. Arthroscopic rotator cuff repair with and without acromioplasty in the treatment of full-thickness rotator cuff tears: a

multicenter, randomized controlled trial. J Bone Joint Surg Am 2011;93(21):1953–60. http://dx.doi.org/10.2106/JBJS.K.00488.

37. Tetteh E, Dhawan A, Bajaj S. A prospective randomized trial of acromioplasty in patients undergoing arthroscopic rotator cuff repair: preliminary results. Presented at the American Orthopaedic Society of Sports Medicine Annual Meeting. San Diego (CA), February 16–19, 2011.

38. Chahal J, Mall N, MacDonald PB, et al. The role of subacromial decompression in patients undergoing arthroscopic repair of full-thickness tears of the rotator cuff: a systematic review and meta-analysis. Arthroscopy 2012;28(5):720–7. http://dx.doi.org/10.1016/j.arthro.2011.11.022.

39. Shin SJ, Oh JH, Chung SW, et al. The efficacy of acromioplasty in the arthroscopic repair of small- to medium-sized rotator cuff tears without acromial spur: prospective comparative study. Arthroscopy 2012;28(5):628–35. http://dx.doi.org/10.1016/j.arthro.2011.10.016.

40. Pedowitz RA, Yamaguchi K, Ahmad CS, et al. Optimizing the management of rotator cuff problems. J Am Acad Orthop Surg 2011;19(6):368–79.

Evaluation and Management of Brachial Plexus Birth Palsy

Joshua M. Abzug, MD[a], Scott H. Kozin, MD[b],*

KEYWORDS

- Brachial plexus • Brachial plexus birth palsy • Nerve injury • Obstetric brachial plexus palsy
- Shoulder dystocia

KEY POINTS

- Brachial plexus birth palsies occur in varying degrees and can have lifelong physical and psychological impact for patients as well as their families.
- The best method for diagnosing and following infants with brachial plexus birth palsy is serial physical examinations.
- Muscular balance about the shoulder is critical for external rotation and internal rotation to promote the development of a normal glenohumeral joint and to perform activities of daily living.
- Assessment of midline function is crucial to assess the amount of internal rotation necessary to perform activities of daily living, such as zippering and buttoning.
- When performing procedures to improve external rotation, it is imperative to make sure midline function is preserved.

INTRODUCTION

Brachial plexus birth palsy is a common injury affecting 1 to 4 children per 1000 live births.[1–3] This incidence seems to be increasing, due to increasing birth weights, despite advancements in obstetric care.[2,3] Fortunately, most affected infants have spontaneous recovery within the first 6 to 8 weeks of life and therefore progress to obtain normal or near normal range of motion and strength.[4,5] However, if substantial recovery is not present by 3 months of age, permanent range of motion limitations, decreased strength, and decreased size and girth of the affected limb will be present.[6]

Only half of infants affected with a brachial plexus birth palsy have at least one known risk factor. These risk factors include large babies (macrosomia), prolonged labor, shoulder dystocia, instrumented delivery (vacuum and/or forceps), multiparous pregnancies, previous deliveries

resulting in brachial plexus birth palsy, gestational diabetes, and fetal distress that is thought to result in relative hypotonia.[3,7–10] In addition, new research has shown that tachysystole, defined as greater than 6 contractions in 10 minutes or one large contraction lasting more than 2 minutes, and the utilization of oxytocin are also risk factors for an infant sustaining a brachial plexus birth palsy (Mehlmann and colleagues, American Academy of Orthopedic Surgery, San Francisco, CA, February 2012). Breech positioning was once thought to be a risk factor, but more recently this notion has been contradicted.[8,9] Protective factors include twin or multiple birth mates and delivery via Cesarean section; however, these factors do not eliminate the risk completely (Box 1).[1,8]

Anatomy

The brachial plexus provides all sensory and motor innervation for the upper extremity. A "normal"

The authors have nothing to disclose.
[a] Department of Orthopedics, University of Maryland Brachial Plexus Clinic, University of Maryland School of Medicine, One Texas Station Court, Suite 300, Timonium, MD 21093, USA; [b] Department of Orthopaedic Surgery, Shriners Hospitals for Children, Temple University, 3551 North Broad Street, Philadelphia, PA 19140, USA
* Corresponding author.
E-mail address: skozin@shrinenet.org

Orthop Clin N Am 45 (2014) 225–232
http://dx.doi.org/10.1016/j.ocl.2013.12.004
0030-5898/14/$ – see front matter © 2014 Elsevier Inc. All rights reserved.

> **Box 1**
> **Risk factors for sustaining a brachial plexus birth palsy**
>
> Large babies (macrosomia)
>
> Prolonged labor
>
> Shoulder dystocia
>
> Instrumented delivery (vacuum and/or forceps)
>
> Multiparous pregnancies
>
> Previous deliveries resulting in brachial plexus birth palsy
>
> Gestational diabetes
>
> Fetal distress that is thought to result in relative hypotonia
>
> Tachysystole (defined as greater than 6 contractions in 10 minutes or one large contraction lasting more than 2 minutes)
>
> Utilization of oxytocin

anatomic pattern is seen in 75% of the population, in which the ventral rami of the C5-T1 nerve roots form the brachial plexus.[11] An additional contribution from the C4 nerve root, known as a prefixed cord, occurs in 22% of the population, whereas a postfixed cord, a contribution from the T2 nerve root, occurs in 1% of the population.[11]

The roots of the brachial plexus combine to form the 3 trunks of the brachial plexus, termed the upper, middle, and lower trunks. Each trunk divides into an anterior and posterior division and these divisions combine to make the cords of the brachial plexus, termed the lateral, posterior, and medial cords, based on their relationship to the axillary artery. The terminal branches of the brachial plexus stem from the cords and consist of the 5 major peripheral nerves in the upper extremity: the axillary, the musculocutaneous, the median, the ulnar, and the radial nerves. Multiple smaller branches arise from the various portions of the plexus, except the divisions, that provide additional amounts of motor and/or sensory innervation.

Diagnosis

Patients with brachial plexus birth palsy are typically diagnosed shortly after birth due to a lack of movement about the shoulder, elbow, wrist, and/or digits. Obtaining a thorough birth history to assess for risk factors as well as to learn the APGAR scores is necessary, because children with brachial plexus birth palsy may have experienced cerebral anoxia during the delivery process. Subsequently, direct visualization of the child will provide substantial information regarding the extent of injury.

The newborn physical examination is diagnostic. Tactile stimulation is used in an attempt to encourage the infant to move the limb. In addition, the neonatal reflexes can be assessed. A sudden extension of the neck causing the shoulders to abduct, the elbows to extend, and the fingers to extend and spread is known as the Moro reflex.[12] Turning the infant's head to the side with the arm and leg extending on the side the head is turned to is known as the asymmetric tonic neck reflex. Usually, the contralateral arm and leg flex, creating a position in which the infant looks like he/she is a fencer. Assessment for Horner syndrome is also performed by looking for ptosis, miosis, and/or anhydrosis, which if present indicates lower root involvement and implies a poor prognosis.[13,14]

The newborn physical examination should also assess, via palpation, for a clavicle or humerus fracture, which may coexist with a brachial plexus birth palsy or cause a pseudopalsy, as the infant resists movement secondary to pain. The presence of spasticity during the examination may indicate the infant having a period of cerebral anoxia during the delivery. Concomitant brachial plexus birth palsy and cerebral palsy can occur in the unfortunate infant.

Once a diagnosis is established, serial examinations are needed to predict recovery and if additional interventions are needed. Ideally, the initial extent of nerve injury is accurately noted so that subsequent recovery can be assessed, as this is crucial when deciding surgical intervention.

Utilization of additional radiologic or electrodiagnostic studies is somewhat controversial because a good physical examination provides the necessary information and none of the modalities can uniformly predict the exact nerve injury pattern. However, radiologic studies that demonstrate nerve root avulsions (preganglionic injuries) are helpful with regard to preoperative planning. Computed tomography myelography and magnetic resonance imaging have greater than 90% true positive rates for determining avulsion injuries correlated at surgery when large diverticula or frank myelomeningoceles are seen.[15] Electrodiagnostic studies, including nerve conduction velocity and needle electromyography, overestimate clinical recovery in the proximal muscles of the shoulder and arm.[16] This incorrect prediction may provide false hope to the parents and delay referral for surgical intervention.

ASSESSMENT TOOLS

The Toronto Test Score was proposed by Michelow and colleagues[14] as a scoring system to determine surgical indications and provide an assessment tool following nerve reconstruction procedures. Five upper extremity functions (shoulder abduction, elbow flexion, wrist extension, digit extension, and thumb extension) are graded on a scale from 0 to 2, where 0 is no function, 1 is partial function, and 2 is normal function. If a child has a combined score of less than 3.5 by 3 months of age or older, the authors think that this is an indication to perform microsurgery.[14]

A more comprehensive score that assesses the entire brachial plexus using 15 different upper extremity movements is termed The Hospital for Sick Children Active Movement Scale or Active Movement Scale. This scoring system uses a score from 0 to 7 and assesses each movement with gravity eliminated and then against gravity.[17]

The most commonly used outcome measure that assesses shoulder function following neonatal brachial plexus palsy is the Modified Mallet system, which consists of 5 categories including global abduction, global external rotation, hand to neck, hand to mouth, and hand to spine. Each category is graded on a scale from 0 to 5, with 0 being not testable and 5 being normal.[18] Because this scale is heavily weighted toward external rotation, Abzug and coworkers[19] added a sixth category, termed hand to belly button or navel, which adds another assessment of internal rotation. Assessing the child's ability to touch their belly button is crucial to understanding whether a child can perform activities of daily living, such as perineal care, zippers, buttons, and so on (**Figs. 1** and **2**).

The Toronto Test Score, the Active Movement Scale, and the modified Mallet system have all been shown to have positive intra- and interobserver reliability with aggregate scores.[20]

CLASSIFICATION

Brachial plexus birth palsies are classified based on which nerve roots are affected. The classic Erb palsy is an injury that involves the C5 and C6 nerve root levels and is the most common injury pattern, accounting for approximately 60% of cases. An extended Erb palsy involves the C5, C6, and C7 nerve roots and accounts for approximately 20% to 30% of cases. When all nerve roots are injured, C5-T1, this is termed a global or total brachial plexus palsy and accounts for 15% to 20% of cases. Injuries isolated to the C8 and T1 nerve roots, termed a Klumpke palsy, are extremely rare, accounting for less than 1% of cases (Gilbert).

Various types of nerve injury can occur for each root level affected, including neuropraxia, axontomesis, neurotmesis, and avulsion. Neuropraxic injuries represent loss of myelin and should obtain complete recovery within several weeks of life. In contrast, neurotmesis and avulsion injuries

require microsurgical procedures to restore function. Axonotomesis injuries may obtain full functional recovery, partial recovery, or no functional recovery depending on the extent of axonal injury sustained.

NONSURGICAL TREATMENT

Initial treatment of all brachial plexus birth palsies that do not coexist with a fracture is passive range of motion. Typically neonatal clavicle and humerus fractures heal within 3 weeks, so therapy is begun at 3 to 4 weeks in these cases. Ensuring the infant has full passive range of motion is critical to prevent contractures and/or joint deformity from occurring. Therefore, exercises should be performed multiple times a day at home with formal therapy sessions used as needed for education and assessment.

Passive range of motion about the shoulder should be performed with the scapula stabilized to maximize the amount of true glenohumeral motion that can occur. In addition, tactile stimulation is important to permit cortical recognition and integration of the affected limb.[9]

SURGICAL TREATMENT
Microsurgery

The timing of microsurgical intervention, when needed, remains one of the most controversial topics surrounding the care of infants with brachial plexus birth palsy. Most authors agree that infants with global plexus palsies and Horner syndrome should undergo microsurgical intervention at approximately 3 months of age[9,21] (Gilbert). However, no consensus is present for the remaining 70% to 80% of patients who have a typical Erb palsy or extended Erb palsy. Some authors advocate microsurgical intervention if no elbow flexion against gravity is present by 3 months of age[22,23] (Gilbert), whereas other authors have noted equivalent functional outcome in infants who regained elbow flexion against gravity between 4 and 6 months of age combined with secondary tendon transfer.[24,25] Furthermore, some authors have advocated waiting as long as 9 months to maximize the possibility of natural history recovery before performing microsurgery.[17] Our preference is to wait until approximately 6 months of age to see if antigravity elbow flexion returns, before performing microsurgery. Further delay yields poorer results, especially with regards to hand function.[26]

Microsurgical reconstruction has had numerous advances over the past decade including the availability of nerve transfers, nerve conduits, and fibrin glue to reapproximate nerve ends.[27] Neuroma

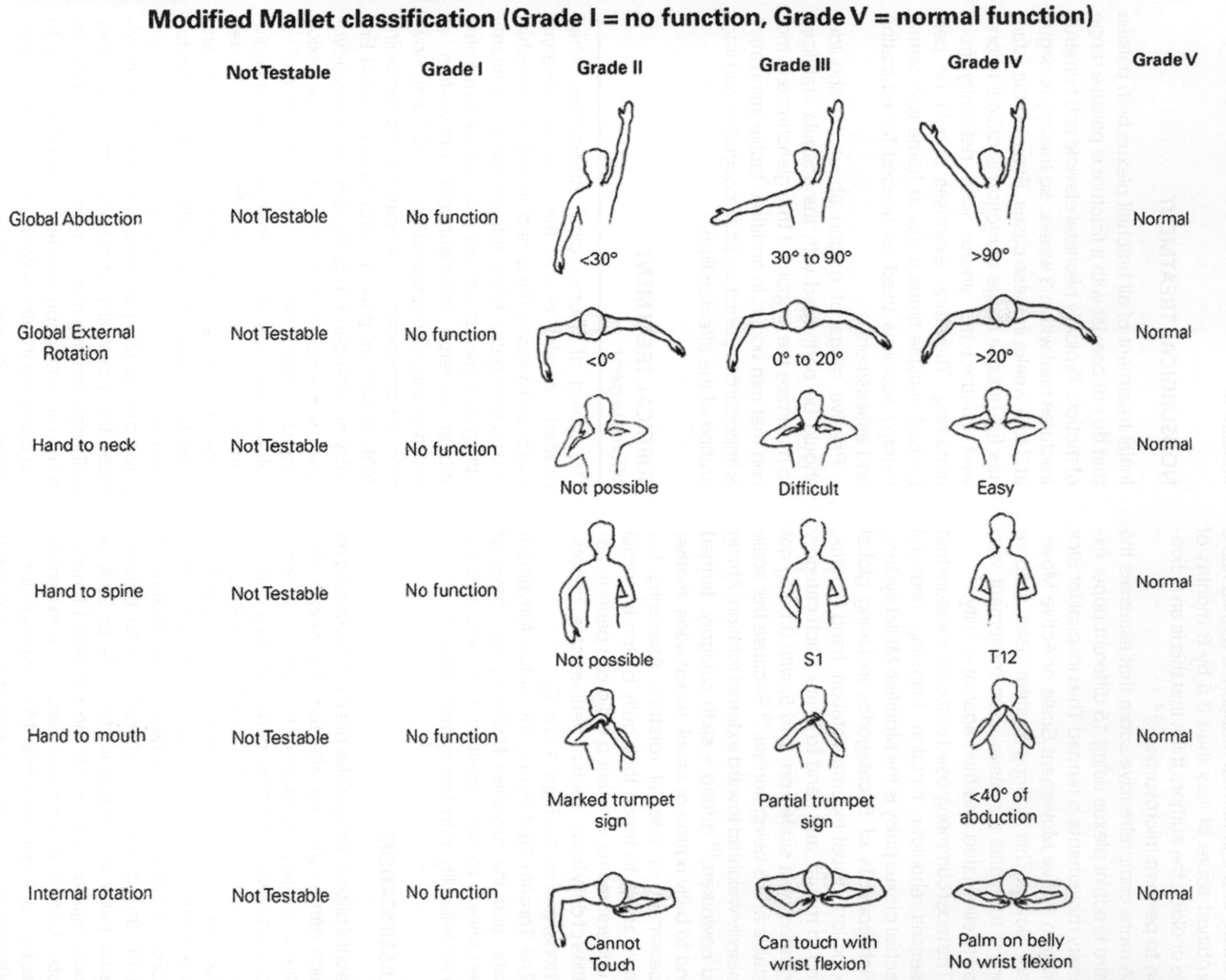

Fig. 1. Modified Mallet classification with additional internal rotational score. (Courtesy of Shriners Hospital for Children, Philadelphia, PA; with permission.)

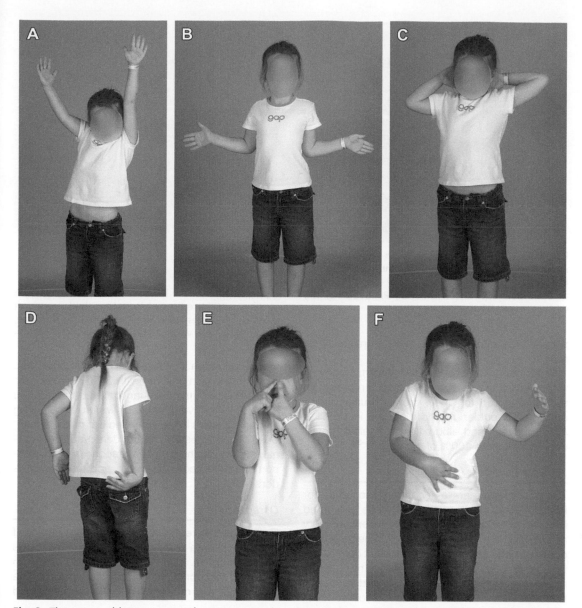

Fig. 2. Three-year-old status post arthroscopic capsular release assessed using Mallet measures. (*A*) Global abduction (grade IV). (*B*) Global external rotation (grade IV). (*C*) Hand to neck (grade IV). (*D*) Hand to spine (grade II). (*E*) Hand to mouth (grade IV). (*F*) Internal rotation (grade III). (*Courtesy of* Shriners Hospital for Children, Philadelphia, PA; with permission.)

resection and nerve grafting still remain the most widely used technique for restoring function after brachial plexus birth palsy; however, nerve transfers are gaining popularity as an addition to nerve grafting or in lieu of nerve grafting. The benefits of a nerve transfer are the avoidance of a donor nerve harvest and the neurorrhaphy is performed close to the motor end plate, which minimizes reinnervation time.

Erb palsy (C5 and C6 root injuries) can be treated by performing a "triple" nerve transfer:

long or lateral head of triceps branch of radial nerve to the axillary nerve, ulnar nerve fasicle of flexor carpi ulnaris to the biceps motor nerve (**Fig. 3**), and spinal accessory nerve to the suprascapular nerve.[28–30] In addition, one can provide more nerve input to the elbow flexors by performing a median nerve transfer, using fascicles to flexor carpi radialis transferred to the musculocutaneous nerve innervation of the brachialis. Other nerve donor transfer options that exist include intercostal nerves,[31] the medial pectoral

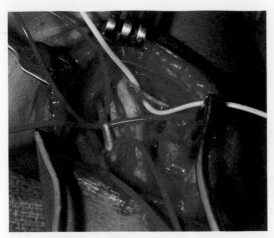

Fig. 3. Isolation of a group fascicle from the ulnar nerve (red loop) for transfer to the musculocutaneous branch to the biceps muscle (yellow loop). (*Courtesy of* Shriners Hospital for Children, Philadelphia, PA; with permission.)

nerve,[32] the phrenic nerve, and contralateral C7 root.[33]

Outcomes of microsurgical reconstruction vary, with the best results noted to occur in reconstructions performed for upper plexus injuries. Good return of shoulder function occurs in 60% to 80% of cases and elbow flexion against gravity occurs in 80% to 100% of cases.[24,34–36]

Tendon Transfers

Tendon transfers are a secondary procedure for brachial plexus birth palsy that can be performed in isolation for incomplete natural history recovery or following a primary microsurgical nerve procedure to further enhance function. Most commonly, tendon transfers are performed about the shoulder region to improve external rotation and abduction to correct the shoulder internal rotation contracture that occurs because of an imbalance between the internal and external rotators. As the shoulder remains in an internally rotated position over time, glenohumeral dysplasia can occur with glenoid retroversion and posterior humeral head subluxation.[9]

Transfer of the latissimus dorsi and teres major tendons to the region of the rotator cuff footprint improves shoulder function (**Fig. 4**) but does not improve any underlying glenohumeral joint dysplasia.[37,38] Improvement of the joint dysplasia requires open or arthroscopic joint reduction.[39–41]

It is important to assess midline function before performing a tendon transfer, because loss of midline function can result in the child's inability to perform activities of daily living such as perineal care and dressing. It has been found that

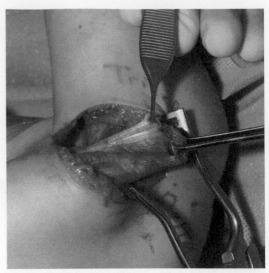

Fig. 4. Transfer of the latissimus dorsi and teres major tendons transferred over triceps into the rotator cuff insertion. (*Courtesy of* Shriners Hospital for Children, Philadelphia, PA; with permission.)

transferring both the latissimus dorsi and the teres major tendons in children with C5-C7 injuries can result in loss of midline function, and therefore, it is best to be very cautious when considering tendon transfers in the extended Erb palsy patient. C5-C7 injuries result in further denervation of internal rotators, such as the lower subscapularis, midportion of the pectoralis major, and the latissimus dorsi muscles.

Osteotomies

Derotational osteotomies are typically performed in older children once glenohumeral dysplasia is present (**Fig. 5**). The osteotomy places the limb in a more functional position but does not improve the overall arc of motion.[19,42–45] This improved

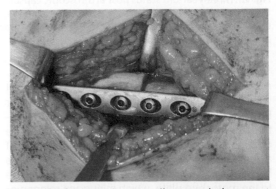

Fig. 5. The humerus is externally rotated; the osteotomy is reduced, and the plate and screws are applied. (*Courtesy of* Shriners Hospital for Children, Philadelphia; with permission.)

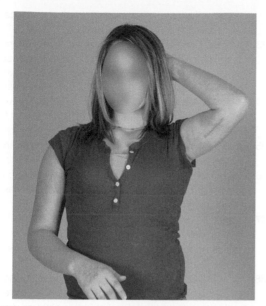

Fig. 6. A 14 year-old female patient after external rotation osteotomy with improved hand to ear and neck. Note the medial location of the scar. (*Courtesy of* Shriners Hospital for Children, Philadelphia, PA; with permission.)

alignment allows the child to flex their elbow to their mouth without bringing their arm away from the body (trumpeter's or horn-blowers sign).[19,44] Either a deltopectoral approach or a medial approach (**Fig. 6**) can be used with a low complication rate reported with both.[9,19]

Recently, glenoid anteversion osteotomies have been recommended, in conjunction with tendon transfers, as another option for the treatment of established severe glenohumeral dysplasia. The short-term results of this are quite promising with improvements noted functionally as well as radiographically.[46]

SUMMARY

Brachial plexus birth palsy continues to be common despite advancements in obstetric care. These injuries can be permanent with lifelong consequences. The diagnosis is made by serial physical examinations without the need for additional advanced modalities. Treatment is begun shortly after birth by performing passive range of motion and tactile stimulation. Microsurgical procedures, tendon transfers, and osteotomies may be recommended to improve function of the child's limb; however, the long-term results of current treatment recommendations remain unknown. Current research focuses on improving functional outcomes by using reliable outcome measures.

REFERENCES

1. Foad SL, Mehlman CT, Ying J. The epidemiology of neonatal brachial plexus palsy in the United States. J Bone Joint Surg Am 2008;90:1258–64.
2. Chauhan SP, Rose CH, Gherman RB, et al. Brachial plexus injury: a 23-year experience from a tertiary center. Am J Obstet Gynecol 2005;192:1795–800.
3. Hoeksma AF, Wolf H, Oei SL. Obstetrical brachial plexus injuries: incidence, natural course and shoulder contracture. Clin Rehabil 2000;14:523–6.
4. Greenwald AG, Schute PC, Shiveley JL. Brachial plexus birth palsy: a 10 year report on the incidence and prognosis. J Pediatr Orthop 1984;4:689–92.
5. Sjoberg I, Erichs K, Bjerre I. Cause and effect of obstetric (neonatal) brachial plexus palsy. Acta Paediatr Scand 1988;77:357–64.
6. Bae DS, Ferretti M, Waters PM. Upper extremity size differences in brachial plexus birth palsy. Hand (N Y) 2008;3:297–303.
7. Van Ouwekerk WJ, van der Slujis JA, Nollet F, et al. Management of obstetric brachial plexus lesions: state of the art and future developments. Childs Nerv Syst 2000;16:638–44.
8. Sibinski M, Snyder M. Obstetric brachial plexus palsy – risk factors and predictors. Ortop Traumatol Rehabil 2007;9:569–76 [in Polish].
9. Waters PM. Obstetric brachial plexus injuries: evaluation and management. J Am Acad Orthop Surg 1997;5:205–14.
10. Hale HB, Bae DS, Waters PM. Current concepts in the management of brachial plexus birth palsy. J Hand Surg Am 2010;35A:322–31.
11. Lee HY, Chung IH, Sir WS, et al. Variations of the ventral rami of the brachial plexus. J Korean Med Sci 1992;7:19–24.
12. Bleck EE. Orthopaedic management in cerebral palsy. Philadelphia: JB Lippincott Co; 1987.
13. Gilbert A, Whitaker I. Obstetrical brachial plexus lesions. J Hand Surg Br 1991;16:489–91.
14. Michelow BJ, Clarke HM, Curtis CG, et al. The natural history of obstetrical brachial plexus palsy. Plast Reconstr Surg 1994;93:675–81.
15. Kawai H, Tsuyuguchi Y, Masada K, et al. Identification of the lesion in brachial plexus injuries with root avulsion: a comprehensive assessment by means of preoperative findings, myelography, surgical exploration and intraoperative diagnosis. Neuro-Orthop 1989;7:15–23.
16. Heise CO, Siqueira MG, Martins RS, et al. Clinical electromyography correlation in infants with obstetric brachial plexopathy. J Hand Surg 2007;32:999–1004.
17. Clarke HM, Curtis CG. An approach to obstetrical brachial plexus injuries. Hand Clin 1995;11:563–81.
18. Gilbert A, Tassin JL. Surgical repair of the brachial plexus in obstetric paralysis. Chirurgie 1984;110: 70–5 [in French].

19. Abzug J, Chafetz R, Gaughan J, et al. Results of global shoulder function after medial derotational humeral osteotomies in brachial plexus birth palsy patients. J Pediatr Orthop 2010;30:469–74.

20. Bae DS, Waters PM, Zurakowski D. Reliability of three classification systems measuring active motion in brachial plexus birth palsy. J Bone Joint Surg Am 2003;85:1733–8.

21. Strombeck C, Krumlinde-Sundholm L, Forssberg H. Functional outcome at 5 years in children with obstetrical brachial plexus palsy with and without microsurgical reconstruction. Dev Med Child Neurol 2000;42:148–57.

22. Bain JR, Dematteo C, Gjertsen D, et al. Navigating the gray zone: a guideline for surgical decision making in obstetrical brachial plexus injuries. J Neurosurg Pediatr 2009;3:173–80.

23. Terzis JK, Kokkalis ZT. Shoulder function following primary axillary nerve reconstruction in obstetrical brachial plexus patients. Plast Reconstr Surg 2008; 122:1457–69.

24. Waters PM. Comparison of the natural history, the outcome of microsurgical repair, and the outcome of operative reconstruction in brachial plexus birth palsy. J Bone Joint Surg Am 1999;81A:649–59.

25. Al-Qattan MM. The outcome of Erb's palsy when the decision to operate is made at 4 months of age. Plast Reconstr Surg 2000;106:1461–5.

26. Chuang DC, Mardini S, Ma HS. Surgical strategy for infant obstetrical brachial plexus palsy: experiences at Chang Gung Memorial Hospital. Plast Reconstr Surg 2005;116:132–42.

27. El-Gammal TA, Fathi NA. Outcomes of surgical treatment of brachial plexus injuries using nerve grafting and nerve transfers. J Reconstr Microsurg 2002;18: 7–15.

28. Bertelli JA, Ghizoni MF. Reconstruction of C5 and C6 brachial plexus avulsion injury by multiple nerve transfers: spinal accessory to supraclavicular, ulnar fascicles to biceps branch, and triceps long or lateral head branch to axillary nerve. J Hand Surg 2004;29A:131–9.

29. Oberlin C, Beal D, Leechavengvongs S, et al. Nerve transfer to biceps muscle using a part of ulnar nerve for C5-6 avulsion of the brachial plexus: anatomical study and report of four cases. J Hand Surg 1994; 19A:232–7.

30. Al-Qattan MM. Oberlin's ulnar nerve transfer to the biceps nerve in Erb's birth palsy. Plast Reconstr Surg 2002;109:405–7.

31. Kawabatta H, Shibata T, Matsui Y, et al. Use of intercostal nerves for neurotization of the musculocutaneous nerve in infants with birth-related brachial plexus palsy. J Neurosurg 2001;94:386–91.

32. Wellons JC, Tubbs RS, Pugh JA, et al. Medial pectoral nerve to musculocutaneous nerve neurotization for the treatment of persistent birth-related brachial plexus palsy: an 11-year institutional experience. J Neurosurg Pediatr 2009;3:348–53.

33. Sammer DM, Kircher MF, Bishop AT, et al. Hemicontralateral C7 transfer in traumatic brachial plexus injuries: outcomes and complications. J Bone Joint Surg Am 2012;94:131–7.

34. Gilbert A. Long-term evaluation of brachial plexus surgery in obstetrical palsy. Hand Clin 1995;11: 583–94.

35. Hentz VR, Meyer RD. Brachial plexus microsurgery in children. Microsurgery 1991;12:175–85.

36. Laurent JP, Lee R, Shenaq S, et al. Neurosurgical correction of upper brachial plexus birth injuries. J Neurosurg 1993;79:197–203.

37. Waters P, Bae D. Effect of tendon transfers and extra-articular soft-tissue balancing on glenohumeral development in brachial plexus birth palsy. J Bone Joint Surg Am 2005;87:320–5.

38. Kozin SH, Chafetz RS, Barus D, et al. Magnetic resonance imaging and clinical findings before and after tendon transfers about the shoulder in children with residual brachial plexus birth palsy. J Shoulder Elbow Surg 2006;15:554–61.

39. Waters P, Bae D. The early effects of tendon transfers and open capsulorrhaphy on glenohumeral deformity in brachial plexus birth palsy. J Bone Joint Surg Am 2008;90:2171–9.

40. Kozin SH, Boardman MJ, Chafetz RS, et al. Arthroscopic treatment of internal rotation contracture and glenohumeral dysplasia in children with brachial plexus birth palsy. J Shoulder Elbow Surg 2010;19:102–10.

41. Pearl ML, Edgerton BW, Kazimiroff PA, et al. Arthroscopic release and latissimus dorsi transfer for shoulder internal rotation contractures and glenohumeral deformity secondary to brachial plexus birth palsy. J Bone Joint Surg Am 2006;88:564–74.

42. Al-Qattan MM. Rotation osteotomy of the humerus for Erb's palsy in children with humeral head deformity. J Hand Surg Am 2002;27:479–83.

43. Kirkos JM, Papdopoulos IA. Treatment of brachial plexus birth palsy secondary to birth injuries: rotational osteotomy of the proximal part of the humerus. J Bone Joint Surg Am 1998;80:1477–83.

44. Ruhmann O, Lipka W, Bohnsack M. External rotation osteotomy of the humerus for treatment of external rotation deficit in palsies. Oper Orthop Traumatol 2008;20:145–56 [in German].

45. Waters PM, Bae DS. The effect of derotational humeral osteotomy on global shoulder function in brachial plexus birth palsy. J Bone Joint Surg Am 2006;88:1035–42.

46. Dodwell E, O'Callaghan J, Anthony A, et al. Combined glenoid anteversion osteotomy and tendon transfers for brachial plexus birth palsy: early outcomes. J Bone Joint Surg Am 2012;94: 2145–52.

Evaluation and Medical Management of Fragility Fractures of the Upper Extremity

Christina J. Gutowski, MD, MPH[a],*, Asif M. Ilyas, MD[b]

KEYWORDS

- Osteoporosis • Fragility fracture • Bone mineral density • DEXA • Bisphosphonates

KEY POINTS

- Osteoporosis is a silent and painless disease until a fracture occurs from a low-energy injury.
- The goal of treatment is early diagnosis and prevention.
- Diagnosis is made through bone mineral density testing, most commonly through dual-emission x-ray absorptiometry (DEXA) scanning.
- The Fracture Risk Algorithm (FRAX) tool (World Health Orgainziation Collaborating Centre for Metabolic Bone Diseases, University of Sheffield, UK) uses clinical grounds to assess one's 10-year fragility fracture risk.
- Prevention is provided through avoiding alcohol and tobacco, performing regular weight-bearing exercises, dietary supplementation, and pharmacologic management when indicated.
- DEXA scanning is indicated in women aged 65 years and older and men aged 70 years and older. Testing can be performed earlier in postmenopausal women of any age or men with higher risk profiles.
- Adequate daily calcium intake consists of at least 1200 mg and vitamin D of 800 to 1000 IU, each per day. Dietary supplementation should be used accordingly.
- Pharmacologic management is indicated in those who have incurred a hip or vertebral fracture or in those with a DEXA scan T-score of less than or equal to −2.5 standard deviations (osteoporosis) at the femoral neck or spine.
- Pharmacologic management is also indicated in those with a DEXA scan T-score of between −1.0 and −2.5 standard deviations (osteopenia) with a FRAX 10-year fracture probability of more than 20%.
- Current Food and Drug Administration–approved pharmacologic agents for osteoporosis prevention and treatment include bisphosphonates, parathyroid hormone, calcitonin, and hormone therapy.

INTRODUCTION AND EPIDEMIOLOGY OF FRAGILITY FRACTURES

Osteoporosis is a silent and painless disease until a fracture occurs with minimal trauma (ie, a fragility fracture) (**Fig. 1**). The mainstay of treatment is detection and prevention. Osteoporosis is endemic in aging patients, with up to 50% of all men and women aged 80 years and older meeting the diagnostic criteria.[1] By definition, osteoporosis is diagnosed and quantified by bone mineral density. However, deficient bone mineral density (BMD) in itself is not as great a burden on patients and the American health care system as its

Disclosures: None.
[a] Department of Orthopaedic Surgery Thomas Jefferson University Hospital, 1025 Walnut Street, Room 516 College Building, Philadelphia, PA 19107, USA; [b] Hand & Upper Extremity Surgery, Rothman Institute, Thomas Jefferson University, 925 Chestnut Street, Philadelphia, PA 19107, USA
* Corresponding author.
E-mail address: gutowski1@gmail.com

Orthop Clin N Am 45 (2014) 233–243
http://dx.doi.org/10.1016/j.ocl.2013.12.005
0030-5898/14/$ – see front matter © 2014 Elsevier Inc. All rights reserved

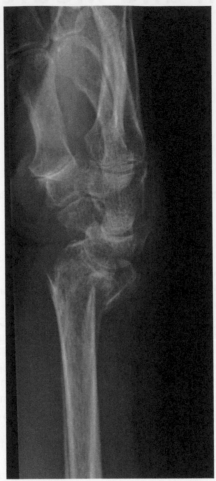

Fig. 1. Distal radius fracture occurring as result of minimal trauma in osteoporotic bone, the definition of a fragility fracture.

manifestation in a fragility fracture because BMD is only a surrogate parameter for an impending fracture (comparable with blood pressure for stroke). Osteoporosis poses a major health problem both clinically and economically because it currently has no cure and leads to an alarming increase in bone's propensity to fracture.

The World Health Organization defines a *fragility fracture* as a fracture caused by injury that would be insufficient to fracture normal bone: the result of reduced compressive and/or torsional strength of bone.[2] These injuries are most often seen in the hip, distal forearm, proximal humerus, or vertebrae (compression) as result of low-energy trauma (ie, a fall from a height of less than 1 m). These low-energy mechanisms represent 53% of all fractures in patients aged 50 years or older and 80% in patients aged 75 years and older.[3] Nearly half of all American women will sustain a fragility fracture in their lifetime, and distal radius fractures are particularly considered to be a harbinger of future

fragility fractures because they are frequently the first to occur as osteoporosis develops.[4] The distal radius fracture is the most frequently diagnosed fracture in women, and the mean age of women with fractures of the distal radius is 64 years old. Women who are 60 years of age with a residual life expectancy of more than 21 years have a 17% chance of incurring a fracture of the distal radius and an 8% chance of incurring a fracture of the proximal humerus.[5]

Risk factors for distal radius fractures include family history of fragility fracture of the hip or distal radius, obesity in men, early menopause in women, and less menopausal discomfort during menstruation.[4] Protective factors have been shown to include moderate daily activity level, late menopause, and hormone replacement therapy. No effect on risk has been noted with body mass index in women, smoking habits, oral contraceptive use, medical comorbidities, education level, visual capacity, hand dominance, or physical activity level described other than *moderate* (which was found to be protective); the lack of impact of these factors is noteworthy because several of them have a significant effect on osteoporosis risk.[6]

THE DEFINITION AND PATHOPHYSIOLOGY OF OSTEOPOROSIS

The World Health Organization defines osteoporosis as a BMD T-score less than −2.5, or a score more than 2.5 standard deviations less than the reference standard (the reference standard often used is the mean score for Caucasian women aged 20–29 years), as measured by dual-emission x-ray absorptiometry (DEXA).[7] This score, thought to represent overall bone strength and subsequent risk of fracture, primarily integrates bone density and bone quality. The features contributing to this include trabecular microarchitecture, intrinsic material properties of bone tissue, and repair of microdamage to bone; all of these features have been shown to suffer as osteoporosis begins to develop.

The theory regarding the underlying process behind osteoporosis is still evolving. The disease involves both bone quality and quantity, rooted largely in unregulated bone remodeling. Remodeling causes transient weakness at areas of resorption but is physiologically necessary to repair areas of microdamage. When occurring in this physiologic capacity, the process is called *targeted remodeling* and is rarely pathologic. If, however, the bone is serving as a calcium reservoir in order to achieve calcium homeostasis in the serum or is being excessively remodeled for reasons other than to repair areas of microdamage, the term *stochastic remodeling* is used and the bone can become weaker over time. Higher remodeling activity leads to both excessive bone resorption by osteoclasts as well as a disproportionately high fraction of bone mass existing as unmineralized collagen matrix, which is weaker and less resistant to bending. In this context, attempts to slow stochastic remodeling are gaining traction as an increasing area of interest in osteoporosis prevention efforts.[8] In addition to the declining quality of tissue, the pathologic process also involves changing bone microarchitecture, as osteoporotic trabeculae decrease in number, size, and thickness. The microhardness of bone, referring to its intrinsic strength, resistance to bending, and toughness, has been shown to be significantly less in osteoporotic tissue as result of these processes.[9]

The relationship between menopause and the onset of osteoporosis has been well established.[6,10] The link is largely based on estrogen's inhibitory effect on osteoclasts. At menopause, occurring at approximately 51 years of age for most women,[7] the relative estrogen deficiency that develops lifts this inhibitory effect, and the increased number, lifespan, and activity of osteoclasts leads to more and deeper bone remodeling sites. Up to 12% of bone mass is lost within the 5 to 7 years following the onset of menopause.[11] Estrogen withdrawal also stimulates T cells to produce cytokines, such as tumor necrosis factor and interleukin-1, which stimulate osteoclast activity and inhibit osteoblasts. The rate of bone remodeling increases, beginning with osteoclastic resorption followed by osteoblastic laying down of new bone collagen matrix to be mineralized. As these steps accelerate, a larger proportion of bone is in the premineralized state, leading to overall weakening. This remodeling rate has been shown to double during early menopause and triple within 10 to 15 years after menopause, leading to profound clinical consequences.

EVALUATION AND INDICATIONS FOR TREATMENT

Osteoporosis screening has become increasingly popular in recent decades, especially since measures to prevent osteoporosis-related fractures now exist. The United States Preventive Services Task Force has established a grade B recommendation that all women aged 65 years and older, without previous known fractures or reasons for secondary osteoporosis, should obtain a DEXA scan of the hip and lumbar spine to establish a baseline BMD score (**Table 1**).[12] The evidence currently does not exist to support the same recommendation for men. If osteoporosis or osteopenia is found on a DEXA scan, some experts also recommend a limited workup for other systemic causes of (secondary) osteoporosis (eg, multiple myeloma, endocrine disorders, malabsorption syndromes, liver disorders, osteomalacia, hyperparathyroidism, and so forth), which can be ruled out by basic blood tests and serum electrophoresis.[13] Baseline calcium and vitamin D levels should also be measured.

Once these studies have been completed, criteria have been established to assess the strength of bone and its subsequent susceptibility to fracture. Tools such as the Fracture Risk Algorithm (FRAX) tool estimates a patient's 10-year risk of sustaining both a hip fracture and major fracture of an upper extremity or vertebral compression based on BMD and weighted clinical risk factors.[13–15] It is based on the theory that although bone mass is a key component of the risk of

Table 1	
World Health Organization's definition of osteoporosis based on BMD testing by DEXA scanning	
Normal	BMD is within 1 standard of deviation of a normal young adult (T-score at −1.0 and more)
Osteopenia	BMD is between 1.0 and 2.5 standard deviation less than a normal young adult (T-score between −1.0 and −2.5)
Osteoporosis	BMD is more than 2.5 standard deviations less than that of a normal young adult (T-score less than −2.5)

Data from Screening for osteoporosis, clinical summary of US Preventive Services Task Force recommendation. Agency for Healthcare Research and Quality. Available at: http://www.uspreventiveservicestaskforce.org/uspstf10/ osteoporosis/osteos.pdf. Accessed September 1, 2013.

fracture, other factors contribute to this risk, including liability to fall, presence of arthritic or skeletal conditions, and so forth, which operate independently of BMD. A comprehensive assessment of all these factors should be used in calculating the global risk of fracture. The input parameters are weighted according to a multivariate algorithmic model built based on meta-analyses studying the clinical impact of each of the risk factors. It is an accessible and self-explanatory questionnaire that is available online for no cost.

Box 1 lists the parameters included in the FRAX tool. Of note, several of these criteria have been shown to influence the risk of fracture in a dose-dependent manner, whereas the available FRAX tool includes them in a binomial (yes/no) capacity. Currently, the tool has not been developed in sufficient detail to accommodate these specific modifications, and the clinician must use his or her judgment when interpreting the fracture probability obtained from the calculation tool. For example, a patient with 3 previous fractures has a higher probability of subsequent fracture than a patient with a history of only one previous fracture, despite the tool's failure to accommodate for this difference.

Importantly, FRAX does make recommendations regarding which patients to treat, provides guidance for clinicians counseling patients with osteoporosis, and provides valuable information on their fracture risk to be used in future treatment decision making. With the ease and availability of information offered by FRAX, the following

Box 1	
Criteria included in the FRAX tool for assessing osteoporosis-related fracture risk	
Age	Rheumatoid arthritis
Sex	>3 Alcohol drinks per day
Race	Secondary osteoporosis
Weight	Smoking status
Height	Parent with hip fracture
Previous fracture	Femoral neck BMD score
Glucocorticoid Use	

Data from World Health Organization Collaborating Centre for Metabolic Bone Diseases, University of Sheffield, United Kingdom. FRAX, WHO Fracture Risk Assessment Tool homepage. Available at: http://www.shef.ac.uk/FRAX/. Accessed January 28, 2013.

question arises: Which patients possess a high enough risk such that intervention is indicated? Each country using FRAX has a different threshold, based on both clinical and economic factors, for treating osteoporosis as a means of fracture prevention. In the United Kingdom, for example, it has been shown to be cost-effective to treat patients with a 7% or more 10-year probability of a major osteoporotic fracture.[16] Additionally, women and men with a prior fragility fracture were candidates for intervention, without even obtaining a BMD test. In the United States, the National Osteoporosis Foundation recommends treatment of patients with a prior hip or vertebral fracture, as well as those with a T-score for BMD of −2.5 (standard deviations) or less than the reference value (**Box 2**).[16] Patients with T-scores within

Box 2
National Osteoporosis Foundation's recommendations of who to treat for osteoporosis
• History of a hip or vertebral fracture
• Osteoporosis on DEXA scanning, defined as a T-score for BMD of −2.5 less than the reference value
• Osteopenia on DEXA scanning, defined as a T-score between −1.0 and −2.5 and a FRAX 10-year probability of 20% or more for major osteoporotic fracture or 3% or more for hip fracture

Data from National Osteoporosis Foundation (NOF). Clinician's guide to prevention and treatment of osteoporosis. Washington (DC): National Osteoporosis Foundation; 2008. Available at: www.nof.org.

1 standard deviation of the expected value are not considered candidates for intervention, and those patients who fall between these T-score parameters are treated when FRAX probabilities are 20% or more for major osteoporotic fracture, or 3% or more for a hip fracture.[17] The World Health Organization recommends the general algorithm found in **Fig. 2**, which includes the calculation of fracture probability with FRAX as a key step, to guide treatment decisions.[16,18]

After sustaining a fragility fracture, a patient's risk of suffering another fracture increases 1.5- to 9.5-fold[19]; a workup for osteoporosis should be undertaken immediately. Surprisingly and unfortunately, the literature suggests that a large proportion of fragility fracture patients still do not obtain a DEXA scan after their injury.[20] Multimodal protocols, such as reflex notification of patients' primary care providers, a prescription for outpatient DEXA scan, and referral to an osteoporosis clinic with or without immediate induction of prophylactic therapy while hospitalized for the fracture, have shown improvement in increasing the diagnosis and treatment of osteoporosis after fracture. Protocols that begin in the hospital, at the time of fracture fixation, have shown superior success rates.[21]

INTERVENTION OPTIONS

Armed with patients' risk stratification information obtained from DEXA scanning and FRAX evaluation, the clinician must determine the extent of therapy to recommend an attempt to slow the development of osteoporosis and reduce the risk of future fracture. General recommendations for maintaining musculoskeletal health during aging include approximately 30 minutes of moderate weight-bearing exercise 3 times per week, which has shown a modest beneficial effect on bone strength in both observational and clinical studies.[22,23] Cessation of smoking and moderation of alcohol consumption (<3 drinks per day)

should also be encouraged. Additionally, patients at an increased risk for falls should begin a fall-reduction program, despite current limitations in available published objective data supporting these protocols.

Vitamin D and Calcium Supplementation

Vitamin D and calcium supplementation are mainstays of osteoporosis prevention and treatment[24] because they are essential for maintenance of bone health throughout life.[24] Vitamin D is a determinant of intestinal calcium absorption and is, therefore, instrumental in maintaining serum calcium homeostasis. The elderly are at a higher risk of low dietary vitamin D intake as well as inadequate skin synthesis of the vitamin because of a lack of sunshine exposure. As vitamin D levels decrease, lower serum calcium levels stimulate parathyroid hormone (PTH) secretion (secondary hyperparathyroidism), which stimulates bone resorption to maintain serum calcium levels in a compensatory fashion. Vitamin D deficiency is defined in the literature as less than the cutoff value of 25 nmol/L. However, PTH-induced bone loss continues to occur above this threshold[25]; therefore, a state of insufficiency is defined as 25 to 50 nmol/L. An increased propensity to falls and fractures is associated with serum 25-hydroxyvitamin D (25[OH]D) levels less than 25 to 30 nmol/L,[26] because vitamin D is critical for normal muscle function, and decreased physical performance secondary to muscle weakness is associated with a level less than 50 nmol/L.[27]

The US National Academy of Sciences defines adequate intake of calcium as 1200 mg/d for men and women aged older than 50 years.[28] Supplementation to achieve daily intake of 1200 to 1500 mg of calcium in combination with more than 800 IU of vitamin D (to increase serum 25 [OH]D levels to greater than 50 nmol/L) has been shown to reduce risk of fractures at any site up

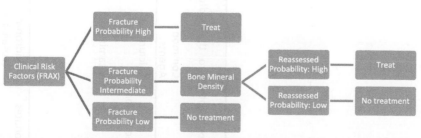

Fig. 2. World Health Organization's algorithm for managing patients at risk for fragility fracture. (*Data from* Kanis JA, McCloskey EV, Johansson H, et al. Development and use of FRAX in osteoporosis. Osteoporos Int 2010;21(Suppl 2):S407–13; and Kanis JA, on behalf of the World Health Organization Scientific Group. Assessment of Osteoporosis at the Primary Healthcare Level. Technical Report. (United Kingdom): WHO Collaborating Center, South Yorkshire: University of Sheffield; 2008.)

Table 2
Pharmacologic options for the medical management of osteoporosis

Class	Common Agents	Mechanism of Action	Indications	Contraindications	Dosage and Route	Frequency
Dietary Supplementation	Calcium	Responsible for bone mineralization and metabolism	Recommended dietary allowances for all individuals	Hypercalcemia, renal disease, parathyroid disorders, bone tumors, and hyperphosphatemia	1200 mg PO	Daily
	Vitamin D	Stimulates bone mineralization and absorption of calcium and phosphorus from the intestines	Additional supplementation required in osteoporosis, patients who sustain fragility fractures, vitamin D deficiency, and hypoparathyroidism		800–1000 IU, PO	Daily
Bisphosphonates	Alendronate (Fosamax) Ibandronate (Boniva) Zoledronate (Reclast)	Increase BMD and reduce the risk of osteoporotic fracture by inhibiting osteoclastic bone resorption	Fragility fracture, DEXA T-score ≤ −2.5 or patients with a T-score between −1.0 and −2.5 with increased risk of fracture based on WHO FRAX screening tool	Hypocalcemia, esophageal abnormalities, poor renal function, and an inability to sit upright for at least 30 min	70 mg PO 2.5 mg PO 5 mg IV	Weekly Daily Yearly

Hormone	Terapeptide (Forteo)	Intermittent stimulation of PTH leads to osteoblastic activation and new bone formation	Postmenopausal women with osteoporosis at high risk of fracture who have failed or are intolerant of other available osteoporosis treatment options	Bony metastases, Paget disease, and prior radiation to the skeleton	20 mcg SC — Daily
	Calcitonin	Inhibits osteoclasts and may increase osteoblast activity, helps regulate calcium metabolism	Osteoporosis, hypercalcemia, and Paget disease	Hypersensitivity to drug class	200 U/Nasal spray — Daily
	Estrogens	Suppress osteoclastic activity and stimulate osteoblasts	Osteoporosis prevention, relief of vasomotor symptoms, and vulvovaginal atrophy associated with menopause	History of myocardial infarction, stroke, breast cancer, undiagnosed vaginal bleeding, DVT, or prior pulmonary embolism	Dosage varies — Varies
Biologics	Denosumab (Prolia)	Monoclonal antibody binds to the receptor activator of nuclear factor-κB ligand and mimics the effect of endogenous osteoprotegerin and inhibits bone resorption	Patients who have failed osteoporosis treatment with calcium and vitamin D supplementation and bisphosphonate therapy	Pregnancy, hypocalcemia, and hypersensitivity reactions to the drug	60 mg SC — 6 mo

Abbreviations: IV, intravenously; PO, by mouth; SC, subcutaneously; WHO, World Health Organization.

to 12%,[24,29] and supplementation is recommended in elderly individuals at risk of being calcium and vitamin D insufficient: those aged older than 70 years, housebound or institutionalized, or with poor dietary intake.[29] Additionally, it has been shown that antiresorptive agents, such as bisphosphonates (discussed later), are more efficacious in the presence of adequate calcium and vitamin D intake.[30,31] Those with known renal or parathyroid disease, hypercalcemia, and bone malignancies must modify their daily intake to avoid dangerous overdose.

Pharmacologic therapies should be considered on an individual-patient basis (**Table 2**). In general, there is strong evidence to support pharmacologic intervention in patients with a 10-year absolute risk of more than 20% for any osteoporotic fracture or a 10-year risk of 3% for a hip fracture.[32,33] The options that currently exist include bisphosphonates, recombinant human PTH, selective estrogen-receptor modulators, and calcitonin. In considering which agent to potentially choose, it is important to consider the risk profile and the individual efficacy of these therapies at reducing the risk of fracture at different anatomic sites because some of these agents have been shown to be effective at one anatomic site but not another.

Bisphosphonates

Bisphosphonates are pyrophosphate analogues with osteoclastic-inhibitory activity, allowing for reduction in the bone turnover rate and a subsequently higher proportion of mineralized bone tissue. Several agents are available, with alendronate (Fosamax), ibandronate (Boniva), risedronate (Actonel), and zoledronic acid (Reclast) being the most commonly used options worldwide.[24] Studied extensively in high-risk women, the various agents have been shown unequivocally to reduce the risk of vertebral fracture; however, not all are equally efficacious in their prevention of upper extremity injury. For example, although alendronate, risedronate, and zoledronic acid have been shown to reduce the risk of nonvertebral fractures significantly in this population (relative risk [RR] 0.84, 0.8, and 0.75, respectively) in the Cochrane review and large clinical trials,[34–36] etidronate (cyclical dosing combined with calcium therapy) has failed to show a similar impact on risk reduction at the hip and nonvertebral sites.[37] It is critical that physicians are aware of these details when counseling patients on options specifically relating to the upper extremity fragility fracture prevention strategy. Adverse effects of bisphosphonates include gastrointestinal (GI) intolerance[37]; self-limited flulike symptoms[40]; and, exceedingly

rarely, osteonecrosis of the jaw (associated with large cumulative doses of these agents in patients with cancer).[38] Recently, evidence has been uncovered suggesting an association between long-term bisphosphonate therapy and the development of stress fractures of the femur; considerable controversy exists currently regarding this possibility.[39,40] Although larger studies must be undertaken to investigate this phenomenon, if it were to exist, this risk must be weighed against the proven protective benefits of bisphosphonate therapy in discussion between physicians and patients.

Teriparatide

Teriparatide (Forteo), a daily injectable synthetic recombinant analogue of the human PTH, has an anabolic effect similar to endogenous PTH. Although chronic elevation of PTH leads to bone resorption, intermittent exposure to PTH stimulates osteoblasts selectively more than osteoclasts. For this reason, once-daily dosing of teriparatide allows for pulsatile increases in the level of this PTH analogue and the resultant increase in bone formation. It has been shown to significantly decrease fracture risk at both vertebral and nonvertebral sites and can be considered a viable option in the prevention of upper extremity fragility fractures, especially indicated in those patients who have either failed bisphosphonate therapy or possess a contraindication to their use.[41] Adverse effects include pain at the injection site, nausea, headache, leg cramps, and mild hypercalcemia. Contraindications include Paget disease and either metastatic disease to the skeleton or prior radiation therapy to the skeleton.

Raloxifene

Although raloxifene (Evista), a selective estrogen-receptor modulator, has been shown in a meta-analysis of 7 trials to reduce the risk of vertebral fractures significantly in postmenopausal women, this protective effect has, unfortunately, not been shown to translate outside the axial skeleton.[42] Mechanistically, its estrogenic activity at bone inhibits osteoclast resorption and allows for maintenance of bone mass despite declining levels of endogenously generated levels as result of menopause. Although a subsequent protective effect at all sites of fracture would be expected, this hypothesis has not been reflected by the available data to date. Estrogens also possess a unique risk profile, including hypercoagulability, and are contraindicated in patients with prior heart attack, stroke, or thrombosis.

Calcitonin

Similar efficacy results have been shown with calcitonin therapy as with raloxifene. Calcitonin is administered as a daily nasal spray; although its significant prevention of vertebral fractures has been proven, its effect has not been shown to occur at other sites despite its known inhibitory effect on osteoclastic function.[43]

Looking Ahead: Biologics

Consistent with many fields of medicine, biologics, agents created by biologic processes, are now available for treating osteoporosis. The most well known of these is denosumab (Prolia), a human monoclonal antibody to receptor activator of nuclear factor-$\kappa\beta$ ligand (RANKL). RANKL is essential to intracellular signal propagation leading to osteoclast differentiation and activation. Denosumab binds and blocks RANKL, effectively inhibiting an osteoclast precursor's ability to differentiate and upregulate in its bone-resorbing action.[44] Early studies show promising results in both increasing BMD and suppression of bone resorption (as measured by resorption byproducts), similar in magnitude to bisphosphonates. One study showed favorable results at the distal radius even stronger than those associated with bisphosphonates. The indications and side-effect profile of these expensive biologic agents must be more rigorously studied, but they represent an exciting and promising effort in prevention against fragility fractures.

SUMMARY

Osteoporosis continues to be a major health condition plaguing the aging population. Despite knowledge of its pathophysiology, our current prevention and treatment methods only modestly affect the natural course of the disease. The major manifestation of osteoporosis, the development of fragility fractures, is a burden both clinically and economically on patients and the nation's health care system, with up to half of all American women sustaining a fragility fracture in their older years. The noteworthy frequency of injuries to the distal radius and proximal humerus should lead upper extremity surgeons to take pause and recognize the magnitude of impact these fractures have on their patient population. Recommended interventions span a spectrum of aggressiveness and have various financial implications; daily calcium and vitamin D supplementation is a cheap and efficacious means to prevent and treat osteoporosis, whereas newer bisphosphonate and hormone agents are much more complex and expensive

but hold great promise in preventing bone loss. Future research into biologics also holds promise, although a full understanding of these agents remains to be developed. It is imperative that physicians, either primary care practitioners or orthopedic surgeons, take initiative in screening and prevention measures for patients as they age. Fragility fractures are manifestations of a condition that has been progressing silently for years in our patients, and the ultimate goal in treating these fractures should be preventing them before they occur.

REFERENCES

1. Looker AC, Orwoll ES, Johnston CC Jr, et al. Prevalence of low femoral bone density in older U.S. adults from NHANES III. J Bone Miner Res 1997; 12:1761–8.
2. WHO guidelines for preclinical evaluation and clinical trials of osteoporosis. Geneva (Switzerland): World Health Organization; 1998. p. 59.
3. Bergstrom U, Bjornstig U, Stenlund H, et al. Fracture mechanisms and fracture pattern in men and women aged 50 years and older: a study of a 12-year population-based injury register, Umea, Sweden. Osteoporos Int 2008;19:1267–73.
4. Mallmin H, Ljunghall S, Persson I, et al. Risk factors for fractures of the distal forearm: a population-based case-control study. Osteoporos Int 1994;49: 298–304.
5. Lauritzen JP, Schwarz P, Lund B, et al. Changing incidence and residual lifetime risk of common osteoporosis-related fractures. Osteoporos Int 1993;3:127–32.
6. Hannan MT, Felson DT, Dawson-Hughes B, et al. Risk factors for longitudinal bone loss in elderly men and women: the Framingham Osteoporosis Study. J Bone Miner Res 2000;15(4):710–20.
7. Armas LA, Recker RR. Pathophysiology of osteoporosis, new mechanical insights. Endocrinol Metab Clin North Am 2012;41:475–86.
8. Sarkar S, Mitlak BH, Wong M, et al. Relationships between bone mineral density and incident vertebral fracture risk with raloxifene therapy. J Bone Miner Res 2002;17(1):1–10.
9. Boivin G, Bala Y, Doublier A, et al. The role of mineralization and organic matrix in the microhardness of bone tissue from controls and osteoporotic patients. Bone 2008;43(3):532–8.
10. Albrand G, Munoz F, Sornay-Rendu E, et al. Independent predictors of all osteoporosis-related fractures in healthy postmenopausal women: the OFELY Study. Bone 2003;32:78–85.
11. Heaney RP, Recker RR, Omaha PD. Menopausal changes in calcium balance performance. Nutr Rev 1983;41(3):86–9.

12. Screening for osteoporosis, clinical summary of US Preventive Services Task Force Recommendation. Agency for Healthcare Research and Quality. Available at: http://www.uspreventiveservicestaskforce.org/uspstf10/ osteoporosis/osteos.pdf. Accessed September 1, 2013.

13. Rahamani P, Morin S. Prevention of osteoporosis-related fractures among postmenopausal women and older men. CMAJ 2009;181(11):815–20.

14. World Health Organization Collaborating Centre for Metabolic Bone Diseases, University of Sheffield, United Kingdom. FRAX, WHO Fracture Risk Assessment Tool homepage. Available at: http://www.shef.ac.uk/FRAX/. Accessed January 28, 2013.

15. Kanis JA, McCloskey EV, Johansson H, et al. Development and use of FRAX in osteoporosis. Osteoporos Int 2010;21(Suppl 2):S407–13.

16. Kanis JA, McCloskey EV, Johansson H, et al, The National Osteoporosis Guideline Group. Case finding for the management of osteoporosis with FRAX®- Assessment and intervention thresholds for the UK. Osteoporos Int 2009;19:1395–408.

17. National Osteoporosis Foundation(NOF). Clinician's guide to prevention and treatment of osteoporosis. Washington (DC): National Osteoporosis Foundation; 2008. Available at: www.nof.org.

18. Kanis JA, on behalf of the World Health Organization Scientific Group. Assessment of osteoporosis at the primary healthcare level. Technical report. (United Kingdom): WHO Collaborating Centre, South Yorkshire: University of Sheffield; 2008.

19. Klotzbuecher CM, Ross PD, Landsman PB, et al. Patients with prior fractures have an increased risk of future fractures: a summary of the literature and statistical synthesis. J Bone Miner Res 2000;15:721–39.

20. Elliot-Gibson V, Bogoch ER, Beaton DE. Practice patterns in the diagnosis and treatment of osteoporosis after a fragility fracture: a systematic review. Osteoporos Int 2004;15:767–78.

21. Edwards BJ, Koval K, Bunta AD, et al. Addressing secondary prevention of osteoporosis in fracture care: follow-up to "own the bone". J Bone Joint Surg Am 2011;93(15):e87 (1–7).

22. Schwab P, Klein RF. Nonpharmacological approaches to improve bone health and reduce osteoporosis. Curr Opin Rheumatol 2008;20:213–7.

23. Park H, Kim KJ, Komatsu T, et al. Effect of combined exercise training on bone, body balance, and gait ability: a randomized controlled study in community-dwelling elderly women. J Bone Miner Metab 2008;26:254–9.

24. Lips P, Bouillon R, Van Schoor NM, et al. Reducing fracture risk with calcium and vitamin D. Clin Endocrinol 2010;73:277–85.

25. Lips P. Vitamin D deficiency and secondary hyperparathyroidism in the elderly: consequences for bone loss and fractures and therapeutic implications. Endocr Rev 2001;22:477–501.

26. Van Schoor NM, Visser M, Pluijim SM, et al. Vitamin D deficiency as a risk factor for osteoporotic fractures. Bone 2008;42:260–6.

27. Wicherts IS, Van Schoor NM, Boeke AJ, et al. Vitamin D status predicts physical performance and its decline in older persons. J Clin Endocrinol Metab 2007;92:2058–65.

28. Yates AA, Schlicker SA, Suitor CW. Dietary reference intakes: the new basis for recommendations for calcium and related nutrients, B vitamins, and choline. J Am Diet Assoc 1998;98:699–706.

29. Tang BM, Eslick GD, Nowson C, et al. Use of calcium or calcium in combination with vitamin D supplementation to prevent fractures and bone loss in people aged 50 years and older: a meta-analysis. Lancet 2007;270:657–66.

30. Ishijima M, Yamanaka M, Sakamoto Y, et al. Vitamin D insufficiency impairs the effect of alendronate for the treatment of osteoporosis in postmenopausal women. J Bone Miner Res 2005;20:S296.

31. Adami S, Giannini S, Bianchi G, et al. Vitamin D status and response to treatment in post-menopausal osteoporosis. Osteoporos Int 2009;20:239–44.

32. Dawson-Hughes B, Tosteson AN, Melton LJ III, et al. Implications of absolute fracture risk assessment for osteoporosis practice guidelines in the USA. Osteoporos Int 2008;19:449–58.

33. Kanis JA, Burlet N, Cooper C, et al. European guidance for the diagnosis and management of osteoporosis in postmenopausal women. Osteoporos Int 2008;19:399–428.

34. Wells GA, Cranney A, Peterson J, et al. Alendronate for the primary and secondary prevention of osteoporotic fractures in postmenopausal women [review]. Cochrane Database Syst Rev 2008;(1):CD001155.

35. Wells GA, Cranney A, Peterson J, et al. Risedronate for the primary and secondary prevention of osteoporotic fractures in postmenopausal women [review]. Cochrane Database Syst Rev 2008;(1):CD004523.

36. Black DM, Delmas PD, Eastell R, et al. Once-yearly zoledronic acid for treatment of postmenopausal osteoporosis. N Engl J Med 2007;356:1809–22.

37. Wells GA, Cranney A, Peterson J, et al. Etidronate for the primary and secondary prevention of osteoporotic fractures in postmenopausal women [review]. Cochrane Database Syst Rev 2008;(1):CD003376.

38. Khosla S, Burr D, Cauley J, et al. Bisphosphonate-associated osteonecrosis of the jaw: report of a task force of the American Society for Bone and Mineral Research. J Bone Miner Res 2007;22:1479–91.

39. Schilcher J, Aspenberg P. Incidence of stress fractures of the femoral shaft in women treated with bisphosphonate. Acta Orthop 2009;80(4):413–5.

40. Black DM, Kelly MP, Genant HK, et al. Bisphosphonates and fractures of the subtrochanteric or diaphyseal femur. N Engl J Med 2010;362:1761–71.

41. Cranney A, Papioannou A, Zytaruk N, et al. Parathyroid hormone for the treatment of osteoporosis: a systematic review. CMAJ 2006;175:52–9.

42. Cranney A, Tugwell P, Zytaruk N, et al. Meta-analysis of therapies for postmenopausal osteoporosis. IV. Meta-analysis of raloxifene for the prevention and treatment of postmenopausal osteoporosis. Endocr Rev 2002;23:524–8.

43. Cranney A, Tugwell P, Zytaruk N, et al. Meta-analysis of therapies for postmenopausal osteoporosis. iv. Meta-analysis of raloxifene for the prevention and treatment of postmenopausal osteoporosis. Endocr Rev 2002;23:540–51.

44. McClung MR, Lewiecki EM, Cohen SB, et al. Denosumab in postmenopausal women with low bone mineral density. N Engl J Med 2006;354:821–31.

Oncology

Preface
Oncology

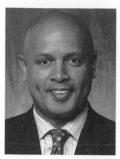

Felasfa M. Wodajo, MD
Editor

In the oncology section of this issue of *Orthopedic Clinics of North America*, we call on our expert authors to discuss the use of fresh frozen allografts in bone and joint reconstruction and the evaluation of soft tissue masses.

In "The Principles and Applications of Fresh Frozen Allografts to Bone and Joint Reconstruction," Dr Luis Aponte-Tinao shares some of the collected wisdom from the Orthopaedic Oncology team at the Italian Hospital of Buenos Aires, Argentina—one of the premier international facilities for bone and joint allograft reconstruction. In the text, he reviews surgical techniques and results of the several types of allograft reconstruction: total and unicondylar osteoarticular allografts, intercalary segmental allografts, and allograft-prosthetic composites. Successful allograft reconstruction requires meticulous surgical technique. While, associated with higher initial failure rates, grafts that survive can provide some of the most gratifying results, particularly in younger patients. Be sure to also check out the detailed video techniques that accompany the article, available online.

In "Nonneoplastic Soft Tissue Masses that Mimic Sarcoma," Dr Matthew Colman reviews the diagnostic basics of soft tissue masses and the findings in several lesions than can erroneously be considered sarcomas. His goal is "to provide additional tools to the clinician to help distinguish common non-neoplastic entities from true sarcomatous tumors." To do this, he first discusses the appropriate use of radiographs, ultrasound, CT, and MRI in the evaluation of soft tissue masses. He then describes the diagnostic findings in a few commonly encountered musculoskeletal conditions, such as hematoma, infection, and ganglion cysts, as well as less common lesions, such as myositis ossificans and arthroplasty-related pseudotumor. Dr Colman recently completed fellowship in musculoskeletal oncology at Harvard University.

Felasfa M. Wodajo, MD
Musculoskeletal Tumor Surgery
Virginia Hospital Center
Arlington, VA 22205, USA

E-mail address:
wodajo@tumors.md

Orthop Clin N Am 45 (2014) xix
http://dx.doi.org/10.1016/j.ocl.2014.01.004
0030-5898/14/$ – see front matter © 2014 Elsevier Inc. All rights reserved.

Non-neoplastic Soft Tissue Masses That Mimic Sarcoma

Matthew W. Colman, MD[a,b,c,]*,
Santiago Lozano-Calderon, MD, PhD[a,b,c],
Kevin A. Raskin, MD[a], Francis J. Hornicek, MD, PhD[a],
Mark Gebhardt, MD[b,c]

KEYWORDS

• Sarcoma • Imitator • Mimic • Soft tissue

KEY POINTS

- Atypical features of soft tissue sarcoma that may be more common in benign imitators include small size, superficial location, soft consistency, painful character, inflammatory or homogeneous signal on axial imaging, or irregular shape.
- Heterogeneous cystic necrosis of a soft tissue mass is an ominous sign and may indicate a malignant neoplastic process.
- Plain radiographs are a valuable adjunct to the evaluation of any soft tissue mass.
- When other diagnostic modalities fail, core needle biopsy at the treating institution is the gold standard for diagnosis.
- The diagnosis should be pursued with repeat needle or open biopsy if initial needle biopsy is unsuccessful.

INTRODUCTION

Soft tissue masses that arise in the extremities can be diagnostically challenging because of the breadth of the differential diagnosis and the nonspecificity of current imaging technology. Although benign tumors are overall much more common than their malignant counterparts,[1,2] the clinician must be aware of and often entertain the possibility of a malignant diagnosis at some stage in the diagnostic pathway.

Fortunately, some masses can be quickly and readily identified before any invasive maneuver because of their characteristic imaging findings. For example, the magnetic resonance imaging (MRI) characteristics of benign lipomatous tumors,

hemangiomas, or giant-cell tumor of tendon sheath are often conclusive enough to allow the clinician to proceed with a treatment algorithm.[3] In other cases in which the diagnosis is not as clear based on imaging, small size (<5 cm) and location superficial to the fascia make the lesion likely enough to be benign such that it can be either observed or excised with little risk to the patient.[4–9]

In most other instances, the mass in question should be presumed sarcomatous until proven otherwise. The goal of this review is to provide additional tools to the clinician to help distinguish common non-neoplastic entities from true sarcomatous tumors. In particular, we review several lesions that have a propensity to mimic sarcoma,

---

Disclosures: No author has any conflicts or disclosures related directly or indirectly to the work in this article.
[a] Department of Orthopedic Surgery, Massachusetts General Hospital, 55 Fruit Street, Yawkey 3B, Boston, MA 02114, USA; [b] Department of Orthopedic Surgery, 330 Brookline Avenue, Boston, MA 02215, USA; [c] Department of Orthopedic Surgery, Boston Children's Hospital, 300 Longwood Avenue, Boston, MA 02115, USA
* Corresponding author. Department of Orthopedic Surgery, Massachusetts General Hospital, 55 Fruit Street, Yawkey 3B, Boston, MA 02114.
E-mail address: matthewcolman@gmail.com

Orthop Clin N Am 45 (2014) 245–255
http://dx.doi.org/10.1016/j.ocl.2013.12.006
0030-5898/14/$ – see front matter © 2014 Elsevier Inc. All rights reserved.

and discuss the diagnostic and treatment approaches that allow safe navigation of a broad differential landscape.

HISTORY AND PHYSICAL

A detailed history and physical examination should be taken, although most factors discovered during this component of the encounter are merely clues and are not pathognomonic for any one condition. Patients may attribute the onset of a mass to a trivial traumatic event, when in fact the two are unrelated, and this should as much as possible be distinguished from conditions that can arise from true traumatic events, such as intramuscular hematoma or mysositis ossificans. The patient should be questioned in detail about the symptoms related to the soft tissue mass, as a painful mass is more consistent with traumatic or inflammatory etiologies than soft tissue sarcoma. Rate of growth of the mass also is important to discover, as progressive growth usually indicates a more aggressive process. This said, certain soft tissue malignancies, such as synovial sarcoma, have been widely reported to remain indolent for long periods. Recent weight loss may give the impression of mass growth when in fact the tissues around the mass have diminished.

The mass itself should be carefully examined. Immobility under the skin indicates a lesion deep to the fascia. A well-defined, firm mass is more typical with sarcoma than other benign conditions, such as vascular malformations that may be less well defined or lipoma, which may be softer. Skin changes, such as cellulitis or puncture wounds, may indicate a deep abscess; telangiectatic vascular changes of the skin are more concerning for malignant neovascularization. Transillumination or a fluid wave may indicate a ganglion or other fluid-filled lesion.

LABORATORY RESULTS

Although most patients with sarcoma have normal laboratory values, a complete blood count (CBC), coagulation studies, and electrolytes may be helpful for the patient being considered for a malignant process. These may uncover hematologic problems, such as lymphoma, hemophilia, or other coagulopathies that can lead to a soft tissue mass. Other laboratory tests, such as inflammatory markers (erythrocyte sedimentation rate [ESR], C-reactive protein [CRP]) can indicate infection or another inflammatory process, but specificity of these studies is low. Creatinine kinase can indicate muscle breakdown, such as

with myositis-spectrum conditions. If the index of suspicion is high, *Bartonella henselae*, *Francisella tularensis*, or *Borrelia burgdorferi* serologies may be sent and can explain multifocal lymphadenopathy.

IMAGING

Plain radiographs should initiate most imaging workups, even when a mass is clearly confined to the soft tissues. Centrifugally progressive or diffuse radiodensity may represent either calcific necrosis of malignancy or true osteoid production of the rare soft tissue osteosarcoma. Conversely, a centripetal ossification pattern progressing from the periphery to the center of the mass over a much faster time course (2–8 weeks) is nearly pathognomonic for myositis ossificans. Phleboliths in the case of vascular malformation may be visualized. Bony reaction or destruction in response to an aggressive soft tissue sarcoma also may be demonstrated.

Ultrasound is a cost-effective, noninvasive imaging modality that may give better insight into the composition of the soft tissue mass. In addition to delineating the size and depth of the lesion, it may effectively demonstrate fluid or blood-product density, and may demonstrate vascular flow through the lesion. These are nonspecific findings, as certain sarcomas also may have large, necrotic, fluid-filled areas or large vessels within the tumor.

Axial imaging is mandatory when the diagnosis cannot be made based on history, examination, and other imaging. MRI with contrast is the gold standard for imaging examination of soft tissue tumors. Content that may be bright on T1-weighted imaging includes fat, gadolinium, melanin, proteinaceous fluid, and old blood products, such as with chronic hematoma. Fat suppression images in comparison with standard T1 sequences are particularly helpful when characterizing T1-bright material. Another helpful finding is peripheral or so-called "rim" enhancement, which indicates uniform fluid content and an absence of central vascularization. Masses with T1 hypointensity/T2 hyperintensity signal profiles that diffusely enhance on postcontrast imaging may represent benign solid tumors or sarcoma. On the other hand, masses that have these characteristics and additionally display central areas of nonenhancement or other heterogeneity due to necrosis are much more worrisome for a malignant process because this indicates either growth-related exhaustion of blood supply to the central parts of the tumor or genetic instability of the oldest malignant tumor cells undergoing apoptosis and necrosis. Finally, one should consider the inflammatory characteristics of the mass along with how well defined the borders are. Although sarcoma can demonstrate perilesional edema,[10–13] this is an atypical finding and lesions with extensive edema in the surrounding tissues are more likely to represent benign processes, such as myositis, myonecrosis, or abscess. Further, sarcomatous tumors are typically round, ovoid, or occasionally slightly lobular in shape. On the other hand, slow-growing benign tumors, such as lipoma or atypical lipomatous tumor, may be irregularly shaped. Other benign entities, such as fibromatosis (extra-abdominal desmoid tumor), may demonstrate infiltration into surrounding tissues, consistent with its benign but locally aggressive nature.

Other local imaging, such as computed tomography (CT) scans, may be helpful in delineating ossification or calcification patterns, as well as detecting subtle changes in surrounding bony architecture. Systemic imaging, such as pulmonary radiographs, pulmonary CT, bone scan, or positron emission spectroscopy, also may be required in certain cases, such as with suspected sarcoma, tuberculosis, lymphoma, or in other condition-specific cases.

BIOPSY

When all other modalities fail to narrow the differential to a specific or definitively benign diagnosis, tissue sampling is required. Although fine-needle aspiration may answer the question of whether or not malignant cells are present and is the standard of care for entities such as pathologic lymph nodes, core needle biopsy is typically preferred for its increased accuracy because of its ability to preserve tissue architecture.[14] This can be done with or without image guidance, and should be targeted ideally to enhancing areas of the mass based on MRI for the highest yield. Open biopsy is also an option, either initially or after failed needle biopsy. Dissection through tissue planes should be avoided, hemostasis should be maintained, incisions should be longitudinal, and should be placed in the distribution of extensile exposures in anticipation of subsequent biopsy tract excision. Open biopsy performed at the presenting as opposed to the treating tertiary center is discouraged.[15] Although false negatives routinely occur given the sampling error involved with biopsy of a heterogeneous mass, the clinician should be aware that false positives can also occur.[14,16] Diagnostic accuracy and safety is enhanced when all members of the treating team, from surgeon to pathologist, are experienced and routinely treat sarcoma or potentially sarcomatous masses.

INFECTION

Soft tissue abscess and other forms of infection can be confused with sarcoma. An acute soft tissue infection may present with clinical characteristics that make the diagnosis straightforward, such as pain, cellulitis, a precipitating puncture wound, or fevers. In addition, edema and inflammatory signal in the surrounding tissues on MRI frequently point toward an infectious or other inflammatory process. Laboratory studies, such as CRP, ESR, or serum white blood cell count may be elevated. However, there are rare cases of sarcoma with inflammatory imaging characteristics, such as inflammatory undifferentiated pleomorphic sarcoma (formerly malignant fibrous histiocytoma or MFH).[13] In addition, a chronic soft tissue abscess may become "walled off" and lose many of its inflammatory imaging characteristics. For these reasons, the entire clinical picture should be considered, and tissue diagnosis via biopsy obtained when there is uncertainty. It is helpful practice to routinely send any biopsy specimen for both permanent pathologic analysis as well as microbiological analysis because of the overlap in appearance between some infectious and neoplastic processes.

One particular infectious process that is commonly mistaken for sarcoma is infectious involvement of lymphoid structures with *B henselae*, otherwise known as "cat scratch disease." This condition presents with unilateral lymphadenopathy that can be mistaken for soft tissue neoplasm. Nearly half the patients presenting with this condition have lymphadenopathy of the unilateral upper extremity, most commonly in the epitrochlear nodal chain. Most report an exposure to the bite or scratch of the common housecat, as this is the longitudinal vector for *Bartonella* species. The definitive diagnosis may be made noninvasively in the appropriate setting with serum *Bartonella* titer measurement. Most patients experience self-limited disease over 4 to 8 weeks and do not require antibiotics. For prolonged or severe involvement, especially in immunocompromised patients, azithromycin is the antibiotic treatment of choice.[17]

Fig. 1 demonstrates the T1 fat-suppressed postgadolinium axial and coronal MR images of a 52-year-old woman who presented with a 2-week history of a distal and medial right arm mass. She had mild tenderness but no systemic signs of illness. Her CBC, ESR, and CRP were within normal limits. An ultrasound-guided core

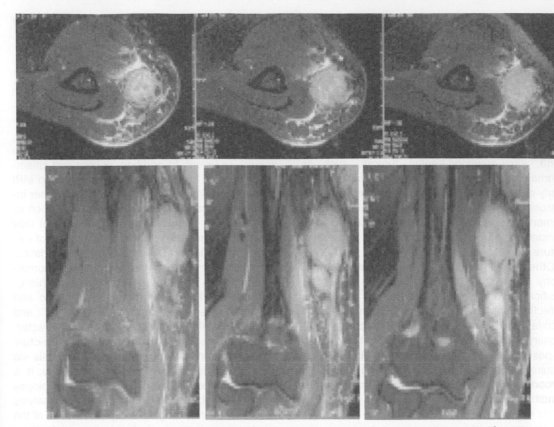

Fig. 1. Axial and coronal T1 fat-suppressed postgadolinium axial and coronal MR images of a 52-year-old woman who presented with a 2-week history of a distal and medial right arm mass. Using serologic testing, the masses were eventually correctly diagnosed as resulting from *B henselae* infection and were treated symptomatically.

needle biopsy demonstrated necrotizing granulomatous lymphadenitis, and follow-up serologies after biopsy demonstrated *B henselae* titers of 1:512 (normal <1:64). She was treated with warm compresses, antipyretics, and analgesics, with spontaneous resolution of symptoms over the next 2 months.

GANGLION CYST

Ganglion cyst is the most common mass of the hand, and when present at the dorsum of the wrist around the scapholunate interval, there is little doubt of the diagnosis.[18] When this mass occurs in other locations or is multiloculated, the diagnosis may be less obvious. Generically, ganglion cysts arise from joints, tendons, bursae, or ligaments. This may be due to degenerative or posttraumatic attenuation of a joint capsule or tendon sheath causing expansion of a fluid-filled capsular sac. However, the pathogenesis is controversial and there may be other mechanisms.[19] The diagnosis is made by a history of fluctuating size, positive transillumination test, ultrasound demonstrating a homogeneous fluid-filled sac originating from a joint, or MRI demonstrating a uniloculated or multiloculated, rim-enhancing fluid-filled sac.[3] Surgical treatment is aimed at marginal excision of the ganglion sac at the base of the stalk from which it emanates.

Fig. 2 demonstrates the axial and sagittal T1 fat-suppressed postgadolinium MRIs of a 67-year-old man who presented with an enlarging proximal lateral leg mass and a dense peroneal nerve palsy. There was a concern for sarcoma from the referring institution, but MRI scans demonstrated the classic appearance of a uniloculated, homogeneous, fluid-filled cyst emanating from the tibia-fibular joint with peripheral rim enhancement. The diagnosis of ganglion cyst was made and the patient underwent open excision of the mass, with resolution of his nerve palsy. The cyst did recur but was eventually successfully treated with further surgical excision and tibia-fibular joint debridement.

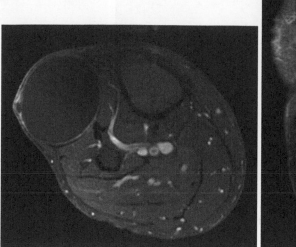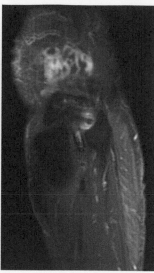

Fig. 2. Axial and sagittal T1 fat-suppressed postgadolinium MR images of a 67-year-old man who presented with an enlarging proximal lateral leg mass and a dense peroneal nerve palsy. The mass was correctly diagnosed as a ganglion cyst based on imaging characteristics, and the diagnosis was confirmed with excisional biopsy.

MYOSITIS OSSIFICANS

Myositis ossificans refers to a heterogeneous group of conditions characterized by inappropriate heterotopic bone formation in extraskeletal locations. Plain radiographs, CT scans, and technetium bone scan are useful imaging modalities to delineate the extent and activity of ossification.[20,21] The term *myositis ossificans circumscripta* (MOC) often refers to the least severe variant, which is nonhereditary, localized, and occurs after trauma or idiopathically in the large muscle groups of the extremities.[22–25] Because of the rapid onset of symptoms and the frequent association with either trivial or no trauma, MOC is frequently confused with a malignant process.

Fig. 3 demonstrates the presenting axial T1 fat-suppressed postgadolinium MRI of a 31-year-old woman with several weeks of a painful left adductor compartment mass. The patient was initially told she likely had a cancerous tumor and was scheduled for needle biopsy. However, plain radiographs taken at the time of presentation to our tertiary center (**Fig. 4**A, 3 weeks) demonstrated a classic peripheral ossification pattern characteristic of MOC. Needle biopsy was deferred, and over the next 9 weeks a rapid centripetal maturation of the ossification pattern was observed (see **Fig. 4**B and C). She eventually underwent elective excision of the mature ossified mass at 9 months from the onset of symptoms.

Myositis ossificans progressiva, also called fibrodysplasia ossificans progressiva, represents the most severe end of the myositis ossificans spectrum of diseases. It is a hereditary, autosomal dominant condition of progressive heterotopic bone formation due to an activating mutation of bone-morphogenetic protein signaling.[26,27] It typically has an onset at a very young age (<10), and progresses in an axial to appendicular, proximal to distal, cephalad to caudad direction.[27] Almost all cases also have congenital malformations of the bilateral great toes. Once the diagnosis is made there is little doubt as to the cause of new bone formation. However, for first presentations and for patients with mild phenotypes, there may be concern for a malignant process.

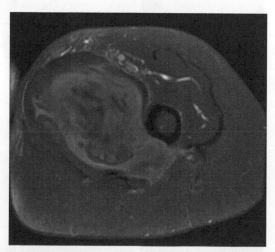

Fig. 3. Axial T1 fat-suppressed postgadolinium MRI of a 31-year-old woman with several weeks of a painful left adductor compartment mass.

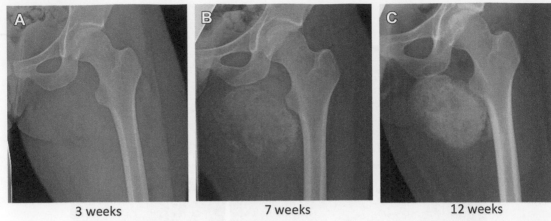

3 weeks   7 weeks   12 weeks

Fig. 4. Plain radiographs of the lesion seen in **Fig. 3** taken at (A) 3 weeks, (B) 7 weeks, and (C) 12 weeks, demonstrating the typical centripetal progression of ossification seen in myositis ossificans.

Figs. 5–7 demonstrate the unilateral lower extremity involvement in a patient initially suspected of extraskeletal osteosarcoma. Although this patient did not have great toe malformations or a family history of heterotopic bone formation, he is presumed to have mild Fibrodysplasia Ossificans Progressiva (FOP)-spectrum findings given the progressive, multifocal involvement of spontaneous or trivial trauma-related heterotopic bone. He also had no evidence for a GNAS mutation on genetic testing, which may be present in other conditions, such as progressive osseous heteroplasia.[28] He was treated symptomatically with surgery avoided given the propensity for recurrent heterotopic ossification in these conditions.

HEMATOMA

Intramuscular hematoma may occur after significant trauma or after more minor trauma in the setting of coagulopathy. In the patient without a very clear history of an inciting event, the diagnosis of intramuscular hematoma should be one of exclusion. Furthermore, coagulopathy alone should not reassure the clinician as to a benign diagnosis. One study reported on 15 tumors that initially presented with the diagnosis of hematoma but were later found histologically to be soft tissue sarcoma.[29] Diagnosis was not straightforward, and was made only by a single needle biopsy in 53% of cases; the remainder required repeat

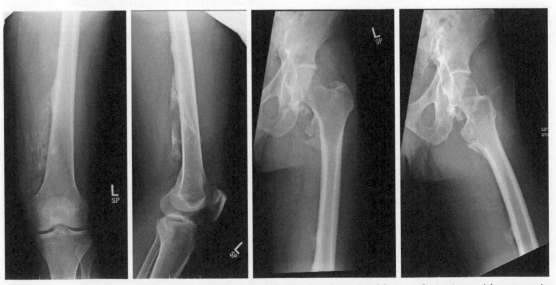

Fig. 5. Anteroposterior and lateral radiographs of the left distal and proximal femur of a patient with progressive multifocal occurrence of spontaneous or trivial trauma-related heterotopic bone formation.

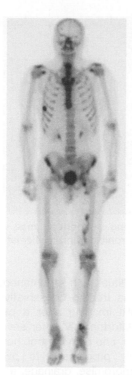

Fig. 6. Bone scintigraphy of the patient, demonstrating multifocal areas of technetium-99 uptake at multiple sites of heterotopic bone formation.

needle or open biopsy to secure the diagnosis. In another study, 5 of 6 soft tissue sarcomas that were initially thought to be hematoma had negative fine-needle aspiration biopsies.[30] For the clinician with any suspicion for a malignant process, repeat image-guided needle biopsy that targets enhancing or solid areas of the mass or open biopsy are useful next steps if an initial biopsy is reported as negative.

Fig. 8 demonstrates the axial T1-weighted, fat-suppressed, postgadolinium and short-tau inversion recovery (STIR) imaging of a 65-year-old man with a right hip mass. Despite the concerning appearance of this lesion, a detailed history revealed a normal coagulation profile and occurrence of a skiing accident 20 years prior. Immediately after his fall, he noticed a small "goose-egg" over the lateral right hip. The mass slowly expanded to approximately 3 to 4 times that size over a 20-year time frame. There was never any accelerated growth. In our evaluation, chest imaging was negative and an ultrasound-guided core needle biopsy was consistent with organized hematoma. Excisional biopsy was eventually performed given the superficial location, and this again was consistent only with chronic organizing hematoma without evidence for malignancy.

DIABETIC MYONECROSIS

Spontaneous infarction of muscle in patients with diabetes is a rare complication of long-standing, uncontrolled, complicated diabetes mellitus, and occurs most commonly in middle-aged women.[31] Anatomically, the necrosis is due to microvascular disease and usually occurs in the thigh. It also may occur in the calf or other locations. Patients present with spontaneous pain, swelling, and often have a palpable mass and the absence of skin changes. Symptoms persist for several weeks, with resolution of the time course of months.

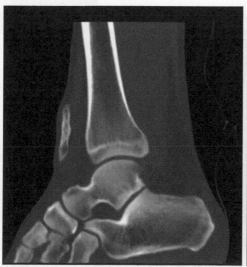
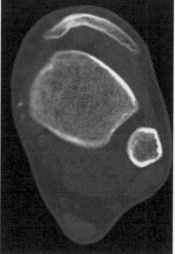

Fig. 7. Selected sagittal and axial CT scan cuts of the left ankle from the patient in **Fig. 5**, demonstrating well-circumscribed extraskeletal heterotopic bone formation.

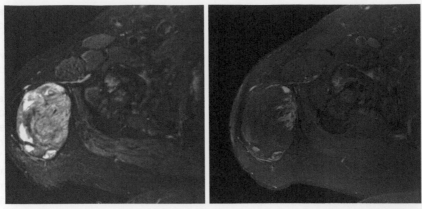

Fig. 8. Axial T1-weighted, fat-suppressed, postgadolinium and STIR imaging of a right hip mass in a 65-year-old man. Core needle and definitive excisional biopsy both demonstrated chronic organizing hematoma.

Creatinine kinase levels may be elevated or may be normal.

Fig. 9 demonstrates the T2 axial and axial/sagittal T1 fat-suppressed postgadolinium contrast images of a 23-year-old woman with 4 weeks of atraumatic left calf pain and poorly controlled type 1 insulin-dependent diabetes mellitus (hemoglobin A1C of 10.2 at presentation). This patient had been sent urgently to our tertiary center with the diagnosis of "calf sarcoma" with a request for biopsy. However, invasive maneuvers were deferred given the diffuse inflammatory appearance on MRI and clinical setting of uncontrolled

diabetes mellitus with spontaneous onset of pain. She was treated conservatively with plan for serial MRI imaging after a period of 2 to 3 months. Unfortunately, after several weeks of rest, elevation, and pain control, her myonecrosis spontaneously progressed to pyomyonecrosis with skin compromise, drainage, and fevers. She required operative debridement and intravenous antibiotics, but ultimately recovered to heal her wound and regained the ability to ambulate independently. Surgical pathology specimens were consistent with acute inflammation and muscle necrosis without evidence for malignancy.

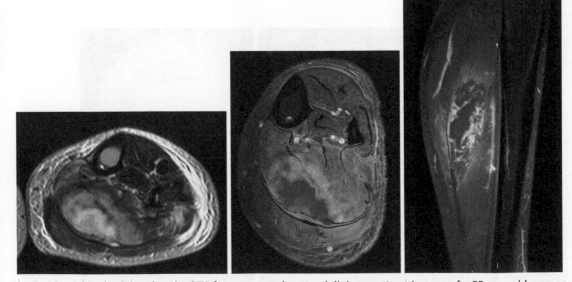

Fig. 9. T2 axial and axial and sagittal T1 fat-suppressed postgadolinium contrast images of a 23-year-old woman with 4 weeks of atraumatic left calf pain and poorly controlled type 1 insulin-dependent diabetes mellitus (hemoglobin A1C of 10.2 at presentation).

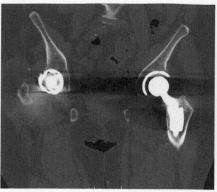
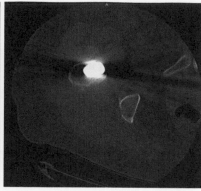

Fig. 10. Coronal and axial CT images of the right hip in an 84-year-old woman 7 years status post conventional total hip arthroplasty with a metal-on-polyethylene bearing. Core needle and excisional biopsy both demonstrated necrosis, histiocytic reaction, and dense perivascular lymphocytic invasion consistent with arthroplasty-related pseudotumor.

ARTHROPLASTY-RELATED PSEUDOTUMOR

Patients who have indwelling hip arthroplasty prostheses may present with large masses that can be concerning for malignancy. This "pseudotumor" phenomenon is most frequently reported in association with metal-on-metal hip arthroplasty bearings, with an overall incidence of approximately 1% in the first 5 years after implantation.[32,33] With advanced imaging, the actual incidence may be much higher.[34] There is some evidence that the cause of the pseudotumor formation is related to local metal-wear debris from superior edge loading, possibly related to excessive inclination angle of the acetabular component.[35] However, there also may be systemic immunologic factors at play, as these patients have higher circulating levels of chromium and cobalt.[36] Pseudotumor formation is possible in other bearing configurations, such as metal-on-polyethylene.[37] The source of wear debris from a metal-on-polyethylene bearing can be from

corrosion at a modular junction, such as the head-neck taper or from neck-acetabular rim impingement. Larger head-neck ratios (although helpful for stability) may increase the incidence of these wear patterns by increasing moment arm and rotational torque stresses.[38]

Histologically, many of these lesions display relatively few actual metal particles. Instead, they often display diffuse perivascular lymphocytic and other cell line infiltrate with areas of necrosis, and the mass effect may become quite large.[39,40] In the appropriate clinical context, the concern for sarcoma should quickly diminish, but tissue biopsy before surgical intervention is advised if there is any uncertainty.

Fig. 10 demonstrates coronal and axial CT images of the right hip in an 84-year-old woman 7 years status post conventional total hip arthroplasty with metal-on-polyethylene bearing and a 36-mm prosthetic head. She had noticed increasing pain and a mass for the year before treatment. A large peritrochanteric mass extending to

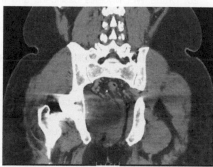
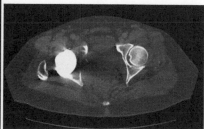

Fig. 11. Coronal and axial CT images of the right hip in a 56-year-old man 8 years status post total hip arthroplasty with a ceramic-on-ceramic bearing. Core needle and excisional biopsy both demonstrated bland foreign body giant cell reaction, macrophage infiltration, and fibrosis, consistent with arthroplasty-related pseudotumor.

the joint capsule is seen. Infectious workup was negative, and a core needle biopsy demonstrated necrotic tissue and histiocytic reaction. Open revision arthroplasty demonstrated significant wear at the neck-head taper junction and histology of the mass showed classic dense lymphocytic perivascular infiltration.

Fig. 11 demonstrates a case of failed ceramic-on-ceramic hip arthroplasty in a 56-year-old man, 8 years status post primary surgery. A large intrapelvic mass compressing the rectum raised the concern for sarcoma. Fortunately, pathology from core needle biopsy and open surgical biopsy at the time of arthroplasty revision demonstrated bland foreign body giant cell reaction, macrophage infiltration, and fibrosis, consistent with wear reaction. At the time of surgery, significant wear was present on the ceramic acetabular insert as well as the neck-head taper junction.

SUMMARY

There exists a wide array of non-neoplastic soft tissue masses that may mimic sarcoma. The clinician should use a systematic approach in evaluating all soft tissue masses that is based on a stepwise consideration of the history and physical examination, laboratory results, and imaging modalities. Some masses may be definitively characterized in this way, but tissue diagnosis via needle or open biopsy at the treating tertiary institution remains the gold standard. Given the repercussions of failure to identify a sarcomatous mass, definitive tissue diagnosis should be obtained when there is any level of diagnostic uncertainty.

REFERENCES

1. Jemal A, Tiwari RC, Murray T, et al. Cancer statistics, 2004. CA Cancer J Clin 2004;54:8–29.
2. Cormier JN, Pollock RE. Soft tissue sarcomas. CA Cancer J Clin 2004;54:94–109.
3. Wu JS, Hochman MG. Soft-tissue tumors and tumor-like lesions: a systematic imaging approach. Radiology 2009;253(2):297–316.
4. Datir A, James SL, Ali K, et al. MRI of soft-tissue masses: the relationship between lesion size, depth, and diagnosis. Clin Radiol 2008;63(4):373–8.
5. Soft tissue sarcoma. In: Edge SB, Byrd DR, Compton CC, et al, editors. AJCC cancer staging manual. 7th edition. New York: Springer; 2010. p. 291–6.
6. Rydholm A. Management of patients with soft tissue tumors: strategy provided at a regional oncology centre. Acta Orthop Scand 1983;203: 13–77.
7. Persson BM, Rydholm A. Soft tissue masses of the locomotor system. A guide to the diagnosis of malignancy. Acta Orthop Scand 1986;57:216–9.
8. Myhre-Jensen O. A consecutive 7-year series of 1331 benign soft tissue tumours. Acta Orthop Scand 1981;52:287–93.
9. Hussein R, Smith MA. Soft tissue sarcomas: are current referral guidelines sufficient? Ann R Coll Surg Engl 2005;87:171–3.
10. Dion E, Forest M, Brasseur JL, et al. Epithelioid sarcoma mimicking abscess: review of the MRI appearances. Skeletal Radiol 2001;30(3):173–7.
11. Kumagai K, Tomita M, Nozaki Y, et al. MRI findings of an inflammatory variant of well-differentiated liposarcoma. Skeletal Radiol 2010;39(5):491–4.
12. Efstathopoulos N, Lazarettos J, Nikolaou V, et al. Inflammatory leiomyosarcoma of the ankle: a case report and review of the literature. J Foot Ankle Surg 2006;45(2):127–30.
13. Kyriakos M, Kempson RL. Inflammatory fibrous histiocytoma, an aggressive and lethal lesion. Cancer 1976;37:1584–606.
14. Kasraeian S, Allison DC, Ahlmann ER, et al. A comparison of fine-needle aspiration, core biopsy, and surgical biopsy in the diagnosis of extremity soft tissue masses. Clin Orthop Relat Res 2010;468(11): 2992–3002.
15. Mankin HJ, Mankin CJ, Simon MA. The hazards of the biopsy, revisited. Members of the Musculoskeletal Tumor Society. J Bone Joint Surg Am 1996; 78(5):656–63.
16. Gupta N, Barwad A, Katamuthu K, et al. Solitary fibrous tumour: a diagnostic challenge for the cytopathologist. Cytopathology 2012;23(4):250–5.
17. Klotz SA, Ianas V, Elliott SP. Cat-scratch disease. Am Fam Physician 2011;83(2):152–5.
18. Gant J, Ruff M, Janz BA. Wrist ganglions. J Hand Surg Am 2011;36(3):510–2.
19. Malghem J, Vandeberg BC, Lebon C, et al. Ganglion cysts of the knee: articular communication revealed by delayed radiography and CT after arthrography. AJR Am J Roentgenol 1998;170:1579–83.
20. Drane WE. Myositis ossificans and the three-phase bone scan. AJR Am J Roentgenol 1984;142(1):179–80.
21. Zeanah WR, Hudson TM. Myositis ossificans: radiologic evaluation of two cases with diagnostic computed tomograms. Clin Orthop Relat Res 1982;(168): 187–91.
22. Wang XL, Malghem J, Parizel1 PM, et al. Myositis ossificans circumscripta—pictorial essay. JBR-BTR 2003;86:278–85.
23. Ackerman LV. Extraosseous localized nonneoplastic bone and cartilage formation (so called myositis ossificans). J Bone Joint Surg Am 1958;40:279–98.
24. Kransdorf MJ, Meis JM, Jelinek JS. Myositis ossificans: MR appearance with radiologic-pathologic correlation. AJR Am J Roentgenol 1991;157:1243–8.

25. De Smet AA, Norris MA, Fisher DR. Magnetic resonance imaging of myositis ossificans: analysis of
seven cases. Skeletal Radiol 1992;21(8):503–7.

26. Kaplan FS, Le Merrer M, Glaser DL, et al. Fibrodysplasia ossificans progressiva. Best Pract Res Clin
Rheumatol 2008;22(1):191–205.

27. Cohen RB, Hahn GV, Tabas JA, et al. The natural
history of heterotopic ossification in patients who
have fibrodysplasia ossificans progressiva. A study
of forty-four patients. J Bone Joint Surg Am 1993;
75(2):215–9.

28. Adegbite NS, Xu M, Kaplan FS, et al. Diagnostic and
mutational spectrum of progressive osseous heteroplasia (POH) and other forms of GNAS-based heterotopic ossification. Am J Med Genet A 2008;
146(14):1788–96.

29. Kontogeorgakos VA, Martinez S, Dodd L, et al.
Extremity soft tissue sarcomas presented as hema-
tomas. Arch Orthop Trauma Surg 2010;130(10):
1209–14.

30. Imaizumi S, Morita T, Ogose A, et al. Soft tissue
sarcoma mimicking chronic hematoma: value of
magnetic resonance imaging in differential diagnosis. J Orthop Sci 2002;7(1):33–7.

31. Umpierrez GE, Stiles RG, Kleinbart J, et al. Diabetic
muscle infarction. Am J Med 1996;101(3):245–50.

32. Pandit H, Glyn-Jones S, McLardy-Smith P, et al.
Pseudotumours associated with metal-on-metal hip
resurfacings. J Bone Joint Surg Br 2008;90:847.

33. Williams DH, Greidanus NV, Masri BA, et al. Prevalence of pseudotumor in asymptomatic patients
after metal-on-metal hip arthroplasty. J Bone Joint
Surg Am 2011;93:2164–71.

34. Liddle AD, Sabah SA, McRobbie D, et al. Pseudotu-
mors in association with well-functioning metal-on-
metal hip prostheses. J Bone Joint Surg Am 2012;
94(4):317–25.

35. Langton DJ, Jameson SS, Joyce TJ, et al. The
effect of component size and orientation on the
concentrations of metal ions after resurfacing
arthroplasty of the hip. J Bone Joint Surg Br 2008;
90:1143.

36. Kwon YM, Glyn-Jones S, Simpson DJ, et al. Analysis
of wear of retrieved metal-on-metal hip resurfacing
implants revised due to pseudotumours. J Bone
Joint Surg Br 2010;92:356.

37. Walsh AJ, Nikolaou VS, Antoniou J. Inflammatory
pseudotumor complicating metal-on-highly cross-
linked polyethylene total hip arthroplasty. J Arthroplasty 2012;27(2):324.e5–8.

38. Cooper HJ, Valle Della CJ, Berger RA, et al. Corrosion at the head-neck taper as a cause for adverse
local tissue reactions after total hip arthroplasty.
J Bone Joint Surg Am 2012;94:1655–61.

39. Willert HG, Buchhorn GH, Fayyazi A, et al. Metal-on
metal bearings and hypersensitivity in patients with
artificial hip joints. A clinical and histomorphological
study. J Bone Joint Surg Am 2005;87:28.

40. Campbell P, Ebramzadeh E, Nelson S, et al. Histo-
logical features of pseudotumor-like tissues from
metal-on-metal hips. Clin Orthop Relat Res 2010;
468(9):2321–7.

The Principles and Applications of Fresh Frozen Allografts to Bone and Joint Reconstruction

Luis A. Aponte-Tinao, MD[a,*], Lucas E. Ritacco, MD[b,c],
Jose I. Albergo, MD[a], Miguel A. Ayerza, MD[a],
D. Luis Muscolo, MD[a], German L. Farfalli, MD[a]

KEYWORDS

- Bone allograft • Massive bone defect • Bone tumor resection • Biologic reconstruction

KEY POINTS

- Fresh frozen allograft is a reconstructive biologic option for large-extremity osseous defects that, if there is not a major complication, are durable for many decades.
- Advantages of this reconstruction are that host ligaments and muscles could be attached to the graft, could be progressively incorporated by the host, and are available for all anatomic sites.
- Disadvantages include host-donor junction complications, deterioration of the joint, possible disease transmission, and that processing techniques, such as radiation, could affect the strength and elastic modulus of the graft.
- Outcome of massive allografts reconstruction could be improved with adequate anatomic matching, infection prevention, modern internal fixation, stable soft tissue reconstructions, and accelerated rehabilitation protocols.

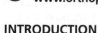

Videos of fresh frozen allografts in bone and joint reconstruction accompany this article at http://www.orthopedic.theclinics.com/

INTRODUCTION

Massive bone loss due to tumor resection,[1–3] high energy trauma,[4,5] uncontrolled infections,[6] or prosthetic revisions[7,8] is a major problem in modern orthopedics centers. Although endoprosthetic reconstruction has improved in recent years, biologic reconstruction is a functional alternative option for large-extremity osseous defects.

Fresh frozen allograft reconstruction has a long history in orthopedics. Since Bauer,[9] who in 1910 described transplantation of bones stored by refrigeration, in a hundred years there had been great advances in fresh frozen allografts. The aim of this article is to describe the outcome and surgical techniques in osteoarticular, intercalary, and allograft-prosthetic composite (APC).

Conflict of Interest: Dr L.A. Aponte-Tinao: Consultant for Stryker Orthopedics; No disclosures (Dr L.E. Ritacco, Dr J.I. Albergo, Dr M.A. Ayerza, Dr D.L. Muscolo, Dr G.L. Farfalli).
[a] Orthopaedic Oncology Service, Department of Orthopedics, Italian Hospital of Buenos Aires, Potosí 4247 (1199), Buenos Aires, Argentina; [b] Department of Orthopedics, Italian Hospital of Buenos Aires, Potosí 4247 (1199), Buenos Aires, Argentina; [c] Virtual Planning and Navigation Unit, Department of Health Informatics, Italian Hospital of Buenos Aires, Buenos Aires, Argentina
* Corresponding author.
E-mail address: luis.aponte@hospitalitaliano.org.ar

orthopedic.theclinics.com

OSTEOARTICULAR ALLOGRAFT
Total Condylar Allograft

This reconstruction is used to replace one side of the joint after major bone loss. This alternative does not sacrifice the contralateral side of the joint and allows the surgeon to reattach the host-donor soft tissues. Although, as with other allograft reconstruction, infection, fracture, and nonunion could be ensue, articular deterioration and joint instability are the 2 complications that are related directly with this type of reconstruction.

Infection is not only related to the allograft reconstruction; others factors such as extensive bone resection with soft tissue loss, duration of surgery, and adjuvant treatments such as chemotherapy and radiotherapy influence the rate of infection. This complication is seen not only in bone allograft reconstruction but also in endoprosthetic reconstructions, with an infection rate of 8.4% in large series.[10] The most extensive series of allograft evaluated for infection reports[11] an incidence of 7.9% of primary infections in 945 patients. In the same series, fracture rates (18%) and nonunion rates (16%) were higher than infection rates. However, an infection complication usually leads to an allograft removal so it is related with a high failure rate.

Fractures of the allografts can be avoided if the allograft is protected with internal fixation for its entire extent. Although in the 1990s the use of plates and screws was reported as increasing the rate of fracture,[12] in recent reports it is the use of intramedullary nails that was related with higher fracture rates and nonunion rates.[13–15] The use of rigid fixation with plates and screws for allograft reconstruction is recommended in most publications.[13–15] The addition of vascularized fibular graft had been advocated as useful; however, in a recent study they do not show significant differences comparing allograft with and without this.[15] Protecting the allograft with intramedullary cement[16] should be avoided in osteoarticular graft due to the possibility of resurfacing the joint with prosthesis in the future.

Nonunion could be avoided if host-donor osteotomy is stabilized with an adequate internal fixation, which is mostly obtained with rigid fixation with compression plates and screws. Chemotherapy had a deleterious effect on allograft reconstruction[17–19]; however, the effect of chemotherapy seems to be a reversible process. When nonunion occurs, it is usually solved with autologous bone graft.

Articular deterioration and joint instability are complications related directly with osteoarticular allografts. Clinicopathologic studies performed in retrieved human allografts found earlier and more advanced degenerative articular cartilage changes in specimens retrieved from patients with an unstable joint than in those from patients with a stable joint.[20] Poor anatomic matching of both size and shape between the host defect and the graft can significantly alter joint kinematics and load distribution, leading to bone resorption or joint degeneration. To have a more accurate size match between the donor and the host, preoperative planning platforms, based on three-dimensional (3D) computed tomography (CT)–derived bone models to choose the best allograft using a virtual bone bank system (Video 1), have been described.[21,22] Bone measures in a 3D virtual environment determined the best match from a bone bank, providing more information to the surgeons for allograft selection before surgery. Longevity of these grafts is also related with the joint stability obtained in surgery with reconstruction of ligaments, tendons, and joint capsule. Deterioration of the joint is accelerated with malalignment of the limb.

Surgical Technique

The surgical technique begins with the proper selection of the graft in preoperative planning (see Video 1). The selected allograft is taken out of its packaging and placed directly in warm solution. After being thawed, the donor bone is cut to the proper length with the use of a navigation system, and soft tissue structures such as cruciate ligaments, collateral ligaments, and posterior capsule are prepared for implantation. With the navigation system the adequate rotation is marked on the graft.

We use an extended anterior-medial approach to the knee, and the extensor mechanism is released when a proximal tibial osteoarticular allograft is performed. The bone tumor is resected with an adequate margin of normal tissue according to preoperative staging studies. All resections are intraarticular and intracompartmental. A transverse osteotomy guided by navigation is used in every case, and the rotation is marked to correlate with one of the allografts. A short anterior six-hole locking compression plate (LCP) is used to reduce the osteotomy. We first apply compression to the osteotomy with 2 cortical screws and then secure the plate with locking screws in the remaining holes. To obtain rigid fixation, a locking compression condylar plate is used on the lateral side of the reconstruction with the goal of obtaining a solid allograft construct by spanning the entire length of the allograft (**Fig. 1**). Soft tissues from the allograft are attached to corresponding host tissues to obtain

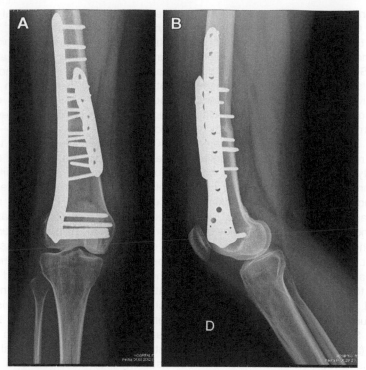

Fig. 1. Anteroposterior (*A*) and lateral (*B*) radiographs of a distal femur osteoarticular allograft made 3 years after implantation with a healed allograft-host junction. Note the short anterior LCP plate and the lateral LCP condylar plate.

the best stability. This reconstruction includes repair of the posterior capsule, anterior and posterior cruciate ligaments, medial and lateral collateral ligaments, and, in tibial allografts, the patellar ligament.

Results

It is difficult to analyze results in an anatomic location with a specific type of reconstruction (such as osteoarticular allograft of the proximal tibia). Usually, the series included multiple locations with the same type of reconstruction (osteoarticular allograft of all locations) or multiple reconstructions of the same location (reconstruction of the distal femur with osteoarticular, intercalary, and composite allografts). Ogilvie and colleagues[23] analyzed 20 osteoarticular allografts (8 distal femur, 6 proximal tibia, 4 proximal humerus, 1 distal radius, and 1 proximal ulna) with a minimum follow-up of 10 years. They found a fracture rate of 45%, degenerative joint disease of 25%, nonunion rate of 20%, and infection of 10%, with a 10-year allograft survival of 45%. Campanacci and colleagues[24] reported 20 osteoarticular allografts (10 distal femur and 10 proximal tibia) in

patients younger than 14 years, with a minimum follow-up of 7 years. The allograft survival at 10 years was 58% in distal femur and 20% in proximal tibia; the failures were related to graft fractures. It is interesting that both reports show allograft fractures as the primary cause of failure. The low allograft survival in this small series could be related because these 2 series included long-term follow-up patients so they are those patients of the beginning of a long learning curve; an extensive series is needed to improve the outcome.

With respect to specific anatomic locations, we have reported on 80 osteoarticular distal femur allografts with a minimum follow-up of 5 years.[25] There were 6 infections and 4 fractures with an allograft survival of 78% at 5 and 10 years of age and the rate of allograft survival without the need of a subsequent knee prosthesis resurfacing was 71% at 5 and 10 years. Toy and colleagues[26] reported 26 osteoarticular distal femur allografts with a minimum follow-up of 8 years. There were 4 infections and 5 fractures with a 5- and 10-year allograft survival rates of 69% and 63%, and 5- and 10-year survival rates of the joint surface of 79% and 65%.

Sixteen osteoarticular proximal tibia allograft were reported by Clohisy and colleagues,[27] with a survival rate of 56% and an average of 90° of active motion of the knee with a good or excellent Musculoskeletal Society Tumor score in 9 patients. Five patients had extension strength in the involved knee equivalent to that in the contralateral knee, 6 had strength that was greater antigravity but less than normal, and 3 had only antigravity strength. Brien and colleagues[28] evaluated 17 proximal tibia reconstructions; they remarked that mild instability and extensor weakness was the most common problem. Hornicek and colleagues[29] reported 38 patients with a proximal tibial osteoarticular allograft with a survival rate of 66%. They did not find significant difference between patients who received chemotherapy and those who did not. Muscolo and colleagues[30] reported 58 proximal tibial osteoarticular allografts with a minimum follow-up of 6 years. Infection was the principal cause of failure (13 patients), with an allograft survival rate of 65% and joint survival rate of 57%. Seventy-two percent of the retained allografts (23 of 32) had some articular deterioration in this series.

Regarding proximal humeral osteoarticular allograft, Gebhardt and colleagues[31] reported 60% of satisfactory results in 20 patients with this reconstruction. Getty and Peabody[32] reported 68% of allograft survival rate in 16 patients but they abandon the routine use of osteoarticular allografts to replace the proximal aspect of the humerus due to high complication rate. DeGroot and colleagues[33] reported 31 patients, of whom 23 were

filled with cement, with a survival of 78% at 5 years. van de Sande and colleagues[34] found that osteoarticular allograft reconstruction of the proximal humerus had higher complication rates (62%) than endoprostheses (21%) and APC (40%). The authors analyzed their series in a recent article,[35] and we found high articular deterioration and fracture rate in proximal humerus osteoarticular allograft.

Osteoarticular allografts of the distal part of the radius replace an articular surface for which prostheses are not readily available. Kocher and colleagues[36] analyzed 24 patients with osteoarticular allografts of the distal radius. The most frequent cause of revision was fracture (4 patients) or wrist pain (2 patients). There were 4 other complications necessitating additional operative management. Of the 16 patients in whom the graft survived, 3 had no functional limitation, 9 reported limitation only with strenuous activities, and 4 had limitations in the ability to perform moderate activities. Bianchi and colleagues[37] reported 12 patients with distal radius osteoarticular allograft. Distal radioulnar joint instability was observed in 8 cases, and subchondral bone alterations and joint narrowing were present in all cases but were painful in only 1 patient. Scoccianti and colleagues[38] reported 17 patients with only one failure due to fracture of the graft. Although no patient reported more than modest nondisabling pain and 6 reported no pain at all, radiographs showed early degenerative changes at the radiocarpal joint in every patient.

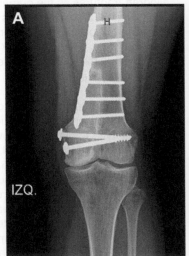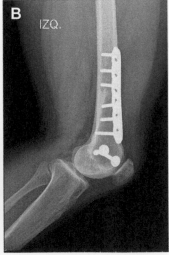

Fig. 2. Anteroposterior (*A*) and lateral (*B*) radiographs of a patient with an osteosarcoma of the medial condyle after reconstruction with a unicondylar medial femur allograft fixed with 2 cancellous screws and a buttress plate.

UNICONDYLAR ALLOGRAFTS

Unicondylar osteoarticular allografts (**Fig. 2**) are used after bone tumor resection[39,40] or trauma bone loss.[4,5] The surgical technique is demanding, but this type of reconstruction is clearly improved with the use of intraoperative navigation assistance.[41] Fracture and nonunion rates are insignificant in this reconstruction due to the metaphyseal location of the reconstruction. The major problem with this reconstruction is degenerative joint disease and instability. These problems could be prevented with appropriate preoperative selection of the allograft in a virtual bone bank and the consequent allograft cut with the use of intraoperative navigation assistance. Although the authors select donors younger than 35 years, the accuracy in size matching between the donor and the host is the most important issue in this allograft. For appropriate selection, the allografts and the host are measured with CT scans. The maximum total width and anteroposterior dimension of the medial and lateral condyles are the more important measures for allograft selection.

Surgical Technique

After proper selection of the allograft, the surgical procedure begins with resection of the lesion, including biopsy scars with appropriate bone and soft tissue margins. The authors use the same exposure described for total condylar osteoarticular allograft to have an adequate exposure of the knee joint. To perform the unicondylar resection 2 perpendicular osteotomies are done. The use of navigation systems clearly improved the accuracy of these osteotomies. It is crucial that the donor bone is cut to the proper length to avoid distal or proximal malposition offset with a consequent varus or valgus deformity of the knee. After the unicondylar allograft is cut to the proper length, it is fixed with 2 cancellous screws with washers. Then an LCP is used to obtain a more rigid fixation and to avoid any fracture in the diaphyseal area. Soft tissues from the allograft are attached to corresponding host tissues to obtain the best stability. This reconstruction includes repair of the posterior capsule in all cases, in lateral unicondylar allografts the anterior cruciate and lateral collateral ligaments and in medial unicondylar allografts the posterior cruciate and medial collateral ligaments.

Results

Muscolo and colleagues[40] reported 40 unicondylar osteoarticular allografts of the knee (29 distal femur and 11 proximal tibia) followed for a mean of 11 years, with a survival rate at 5 years of 85%.

There were 6 failures due to 2 local recurrences, 2 infections, 1 fracture, and 1 massive resorption. Bianchi and colleagues[39] reported 12 unicondylar osteoarticular allograft (9 distal femur and 3 proximal tibia) with a minimum follow-up of 4 years. They had 2 failures, and the remaining patients had mild or severe degenerative changes.

INTERCALARY ALLOGRAFTS
Allograft Arthrodesis

Massive allograft arthrodesis is a salvage procedure reserved in cases when a great loss of soft tissue is present such as after extra-articular tumor resection or failed previous reconstruction with complete loss of muscle function involved in the joint movement.

Benevenia and colleagues[42] reported on 25 patients, 11 of whom had nononcological complications following intercalary allograft arthrodesis of the knee. Weiner and colleagues[43] reported 18% of nonunion in 39 patients who had an allograft arthrodesis after resection of a tumor around the knee. Mankin and colleagues[3] reported that only 3% had an excellent result and 51% had a good result, according to their scoring system after reviewing 71 patients who had an allograft arthrodesis. Donati and colleagues[44] reported a two-center study of 92 patients with knee arthrodesis. They found that complications were greater (infection 20%, fracture 25%, nonunion 44%) and outcome less successful, in comparison with other allograft reconstructions. This is due to the greater soft-tissue resection after extra-articular resection. In addition, the allografts implanted in replacement of the knee may not be strong enough to resist high rotational forces ordinarily acting on the knee.

Intercalary Segmental Allografts

Intercalary segmental allograft avoids complications associated with osteoarticular allograft, such as degenerative joint disease or instability. The functional results are better than osteoarticular or allograft composite,[13–15,45] with lower infection rate (6%).[11] The main complications in this type of reconstruction are mechanical such as fracture and nonunion. These 2 complications could be avoided with a rigid internal fixation with plates and screws. Frisoni and colleagues[15] analyzed factors that affected outcome in intercalary segmental allograft and found that the use of intramedullary nails had an adverse relationship with fracture and nonunion. Although this reconstruction combined with a vascularized fibular graft diminished the rate of nonunion, they found no differences in fracture rates. The authors found[14] similar results in intercalary femoral allograft with a fracture rate of 17%, leading to replacement of the graft in all cases except one. In the tibia, however, we found that the fracture rate was lower (11%) with intercalary allograft, and all these fractures were treated with autologous graft without failure of the original allograft.[45] These differences between femur and tibia allografts could be explained by the presence of the fibula, which could help to transmit load to the ankle joint. Although Ortiz-Cruz and colleagues[46] reported that they did not find any differences in nonunion in diaphyseal or metaphyseal bone, or with different internal fixation, Cara and colleagues[47] and Muscolo and colleagues[13] reported nonunion mainly in diaphyseal osteotomies. In the last study,[13] the nonunion rate for diaphyseal junctions was higher (15%) than the rate for metaphyseal ones (2%).

Surgical Technique

The surgical procedure begins with resection of the lesion, including biopsy scars with appropriate bone and soft tissue margins (Video 2). The surgical resection could be performed more accurately assisted by computer navigation. After being thawed in a warm solution a fresh deep-frozen allograft segment, sized to fit the bone defect, is cut to the proper length. All allograft-host junctions are made with a transverse osteotomy. Each osteotomy is first stabilized with a short LCP plate; this simplifies the reduction of each osteotomy. After compression of the host donor junction with at least 2 cortical screws, we placed locking screws. When both osteotomies are secured the authors placed a third long plate to achieve a more rigid fixation and protect the whole graft (**Fig. 3**).

The use of intercalary allografts in the last 2 decades has increased with advances in imaging techniques that allow for more accurate transepiphyseal osteotomies with epiphyseal preservation.[48–54] The epiphysis can then be fixed to intercalary segmental allografts, maintaining the articular cartilage and joint ligaments of the patient. These osteotomies usually heal without complication, allowing limb stability and normal joints motion. In recent years,[55,56] the use of navigation was reported to perform these osteotomies more accurately.

The surgical technique after transepiphyseal osteotomies differs in that only cancellous screws are used for fixation at the epiphyseal host-donor junctions when a thin epiphyseal segment is saved (Videos 3 and 4). However, the authors recommend placing at least 1 or 2 screws of the long

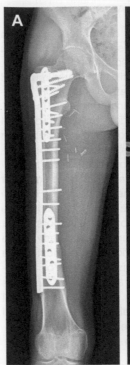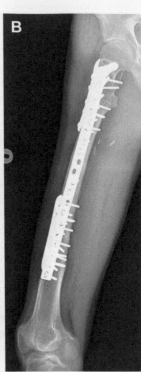

Fig. 3. Anteroposterior (A) and lateral (B) radiographs 3 years after resection of an osteosarcoma and reconstruction with a femur intercalary allograft. Note both osteotomies are stabilized with 2 anterior short plates and a long plate cover the whole graft.

plate in the host epiphysis to protect the construct when possible (**Fig. 4**). They found that although this junction healed quickly, the metaphyseal area is the one that suffers most of the allograft fractures.

Hemicylindrical Intercalary Allografts

Hemicylindrical intercalary allografts were originally described after resection of low-grade surface tumors (**Fig. 5**)[57,58] or to reconstruct the cortical window after intralesional curettage of a benign lesion (Video 5).[59,60] In recent years, this type of reconstruction had been described after multiplanar osteotomies to save the joint with[61,62] or without[63,64] the assistance of intraoperative navigation.

Combining fragmented bone morselized allograft and hemicylindrical intercalary allograft after intralesional curettage of benign aggressive tumors had been described (see Video 5),[59,60] which allows immediate partial weight bearing and maintained the fragmented allografts packed in place. Deijkers and colleagues[57] performed 22 hemicortical procedures in selected patients with low-grade sarcomas. All allografts incorporated completely,

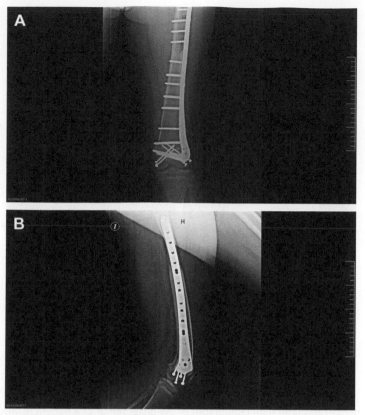

Fig. 4. Anteroposterior (*A*) and lateral (*B*) radiographs 5 years after transepiphyseal resection of an osteosarcoma located at the distal femur and reconstruction with an intercalary allograft that shows healing of graft-host junction.

and there were no fractures or infections; however, wide resection margins were obtained in 19 patients. In this complex type of resection, navigation is clearly an advantage as shown in 2 recent reports.[61,62] This technology allows proper free margins and the allograft is easily cut to fit the defect.

ALLOGRAFT-PROSTHETIC COMPOSITES

The combination of an allograft and a prosthesis (composite biologic implant) had the advantage of reinsertion of soft tissue structures in the joint providing stability without the need of adequate size-match between the donor and the host. Originally it was almost always performed for bone tumor resections,[65] but in the last decade it is increasingly used after failed revision arthroplasties.[66,67] Allografts provide more stability and consequently improve function in comparison with endoposthetic replacement[68,69] due to the ability of tendon reinsertion such as abductor muscles in the hip, extensor mechanism in the proximal tibia, and rotator cuff in the shoulder.

Surgical Technique

Once the surgical procedure begins, simultaneously while tumor resection is performed, the allograft is prepared on a separate clean table and the cuts are performed according to the prosthesis guide (Video 6). The authors recommend that the prosthesis is cemented to the allograft and the stem be secured to the host-bone uncemented. If rotational instability after the stem is placed, the composite must be fixed to the host bone with plate and screws. For proximal femur and distal femur APCs, the authors recommend to always additionally fix with a plate and screws (**Fig. 6**, see Video 6). However, this is not always necessary in the proximal humerus and proximal tibia. The final step of the reconstruction consists of reattachment of the host tendons to the allografts.

Results

Proximal femur allograft composite prosthesis is the more extensively reported in the literature (**Fig. 7**). Zehr and colleagues[70] compared 18 megaprostheses with 18 APC following resection of the

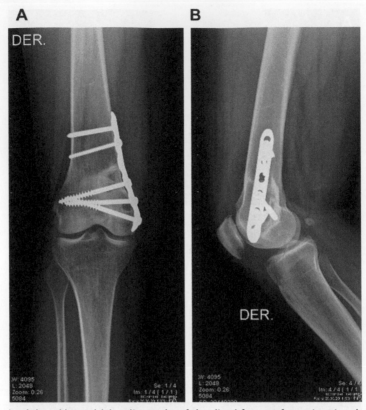

Fig. 5. Anteroposterior (*A*) and lateral (*B*) radiographs of the distal femur of a patient in whom a hemicylindrical allograft was performed after resection of the low-grade malignant bone tumor and stabilized with a plate.

proximal part of the femur, with a 10-year survival of 58% in the megaprosthesis group and 76% in the APC group. They found no significant differences in clinical function or in the longevity of the reconstructions but instability was found in 28% of the megaprostheses. Farid and colleagues[69] compared results between 52 endoprosthesis and 20 APC and found no differences in survival (86% at 10 years for both groups). However, the median hip abductor strength was greater for APC reconstructions. Langlais and colleagues[71] had a survival at 10 years of composite prostheses of 81% compared with only 65% for megaprostheses with better functional results in the APC group. Benedetti and colleagues[68] compared the gait between endoprosthesis reconstructions and APC of the proximal femur and found that direct fixation of the muscles to the allograft provide a more efficient muscle recovery. Muscolo and colleagues[72] found better gait with direct tendon-to-tendon suture of the abductor mechanism than trochanteric osteotomy. Biau and colleagues[73] showed worse resorption in gamma radiation allografts than fresh frozen allografts, so they recommend fresh frozen allografts for massive reconstructions.

Farfalli and colleagues[74] compared 50 knee APCs performed with nonconstrained revision knee prosthesis with 36 APCs performed with a constrained prosthesis and found similar survival rate and functional scores in both groups. However, they found that distal femur APCs survival was worse (73% at 5 years and 48% at 10 years) than proximal tibial APCs (75% at 5 years and 10 years). They recommend long stem fixation to avoid fractures. The same recommendation was made by Gilbert and colleagues.[75] Donati and colleagues[76] had similar survival at 5 years and 10 years for proximal tibia APC, but Biau and colleagues[77] described poor results for proximal tibial reconstruction sterilized by gamma radiation.

Reconstructions with APC in the proximal humerus show no differences regarding complications or survival with other methods[78] but is preferred over osteoarticular allograft because it avoids the risk of articular fractures and collapse.[14] In the last years,[79] the use of reverse shoulder prosthesis-allograft composite had been described but long-term studies are needed to evaluate the longevity of this construct. Atrophy of the deltoid muscle is the major concern after this reconstruction.

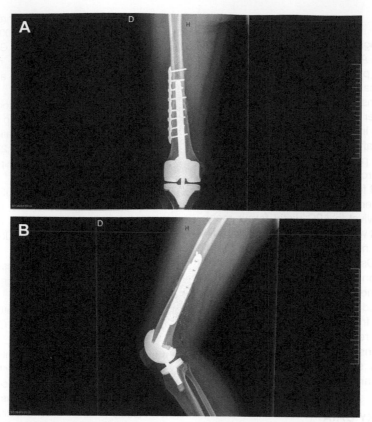

Fig. 6. Anteroposterior (*A*) and lateral (*B*) radiographs of a patient in whom an allograft-prosthetic composite of the distal femur was performed after resection of an osteosarcoma. The long stem protects the allograft with the addition of an LCP plate.

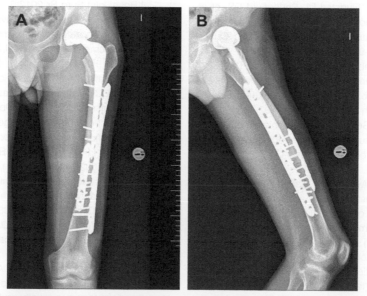

Fig. 7. Anteroposterior (*A*) and lateral (*B*) radiographs of a patient 3 years after resection of an osteosarcoma of the proximal femur in whom an allograft-prosthetic composite was performed. Note the short anterior plate and the lateral long plate to decrease the risk of fracture.

SUMMARY

Fresh frozen allografts have an established and proven outcome. Although endoprosthetic reconstruction is the preferred reconstructive option for large bone massive defects in most centers, there are situations that bone allograft reconstruction clearly better restore normal anatomy and function, such as intercalary segmental and hemicylindrical allografts. APC reconstruction is the current choice in proximal humerus, elbow, proximal femur, and proximal tibia reconstructions. Osteoarticular distal femur and distal radius allograft are preferred over APC reconstruction, the first because the survival in APC distal femur reconstruction showed worst results and in distal radius because there is not adequate prosthesis for this reconstruction. Osteoarticular allograft are more demanding reconstructions that need a long learning curve and a reliable modern bone bank to provide the adequate graft for each patient. However, fresh frozen allograft reconstructions allow bone stock restoration and host joint preservation in situations where endoprosthetic reconstructions would sacrifice normal host bone or uncompromised articular surface.

SUPPLEMENTARY DATA

Videos related to this article can be found online at http://dx.doi.org/10.1016/j.ocl.2013.12.008.

REFERENCES

1. Gebhardt MC, Flugstad DI, Springfield DS, et al. The use of bone allografts for limb salvage in high-grade extremity osteosarcoma. Clin Orthop 1991;270:181–96.
2. Mankin HJ, Gebhardt MC, Tomford WW. The use of frozen cadaveric allografts in the management of patients with bone tumors of the extremities. Orthop Clin North Am 1987;18:275–89.
3. Mankin HJ, Gebhardt MC, Jennings LC, et al. Long-term results of allograft replacement in the management of bone tumors. Clin Orthop 1996; 324:86–97.
4. Muscolo DL, Ayerza MA, Aponte Tinao LA, et al. Distal femur osteoarticular allograft reconstruction after grade III open fractures in pediatric patients. J Orthop Trauma 2004;18(5):312–5.
5. Lee JH, Wang SI, Choi HR, et al. Unicondylarosteoarticular allograft reconstruction of the distal femur in a patient with a traumatic osteoarticular defect of the lateral femoral condyle. Knee Surg Sports Traumatol Arthrosc 2011;19(4):556–8.
6. Muscolo DL, Carbo L, Aponte-Tinao LA, et al. Massive bone loss from fungal infection after anterior cruciate ligament arthroscopic reconstruction. Clin Orthop Relat Res 2009;467(9):2420–5.
7. Gitelis S, Heligman D, Quill G, et al. The use of large allografts for tumor reconstruction and salvage of the failed total hip arthroplasty. Clin Orthop 1988;231:62–70.
8. Rogers BA, Sternheim A, De Iorio M, et al. Proximal femoral allograft in revision hip surgery with severe femoral bone loss: a systematic review and meta-analysis. J Arthroplasty 2012;27(6):829–36.
9. Bauer H. Ueberknochentransplantation. Zentralbl Chir 1910;37:20–1.
10. Henderson ER, Groundland JS, Pala E, et al. Failure mode classification for tumor endoprostheses: retrospective review of five institutions and a literature review. J Bone Joint Surg Am 2011; 93(5):418–29.
11. Mankin HJ, Hornicek FJ, Raskin KA. Infection in massive bone allografts. Clin Orthop Relat Res 2005;(432):210–6.
12. Sorger JI, Hornicek FJ, Zavatta M, et al. Allograft fractures revisited. Clin Orthop Relat Res 2001;(382):66–74.
13. Muscolo DL, Ayerza MA, Aponte-Tinao L, et al. Intercalary femur and tibia segmental allografts provide an acceptable alternative in reconstructing tumor resections. Clin Orthop Relat Res 2004;(426):97–102.
14. Aponte-Tinao L, Farfalli GL, Ritacco LE, et al. Intercalary femur allografts are an acceptable alternative after tumor resection. Clin Orthop Relat Res 2012;470(3):728–34.
15. Frisoni T, Cevolani L, Giorgini A, et al. Factors affecting outcome of massive intercalary bone allografts in the treatment of tumours of the femur. J Bone Joint Surg Br 2012;94(6):836–41.
16. Gerrand CH, Griffin AM, Davis AM, et al. Large segment allograft survival is improved with intramedullary cement. J Surg Oncol 2003;84:198–208.
17. Hornicek FJ, Gebhardt MC, Tomford WW, et al. Factors affecting nonunion of the allograft-host junction. Clin Orthop Relat Res 2001;(382):87–98.
18. Friedlander GE, Tross RB, Doganis AC, et al. Effects of chemotherapeutic agents on bone. Short-term methotrexate and doxorubicin (Adriamycin) treatment in a rat model. J Bone Joint Surg Am 1984;66A:602–7.
19. Hazan EJ, Hornicek FJ, Tomford WW, et al. The effect of adjuvant chemotherapy on osteoarticular allografts. Clin Orthop 2001;385:176–81.
20. Enneking WF, Campanacci DA. Retrieved human allografts. A clinicopathological study. J Bone Joint Surg Am 2001;83A:971–86.
21. Ritacco LE, Espinoza Orías AA, Aponte-Tinao L, et al. Three-dimensional morphometric analysis of the distal femur: a validity method for allograft selection using a virtual bone bank. Stud Health Technol Inform 2010;160(Pt 2):1287–90.

22. Ritacco LE, Seiler C, Farfalli GL, et al. Validity of an automatic measure protocol in distal femur for allograft selection from a three-dimensional virtual bone bank system. Cell Tissue Bank 2013;14(2):213–20.

23. Ogilvie CM, Crawford EA, Hosalkar HS, et al. Long-term results for limb salvage with osteoarticular allograft reconstruction. Clin Orthop Relat Res 2009;467(10):2685–90.

24. Campanacci L, Manfrini M, Colangeli M, et al. Long-term results in children with massive bone osteoarticular allografts of the knee for high-grade osteosarcoma. J Pediatr Orthop 2010;30(8):919–27.

25. Muscolo DL, Ayerza MA, Aponte-Tinao LA, et al. The use of distal femoral osteoarticular allograft in limb salvage surgery. J Bone Joint Surg Am 2005;87(11):2449–55.

26. Toy PC, White JR, Scarborough MT, et al. Distal femoral osteoarticular allografts: long-term survival, but frequent complications. Clin Orthop Relat Res 2010;468(11):2914–23.

27. Clohisy DR, Mankin HJ. Osteoarticular allografts for reconstruction after resection of a musculoskeletal tumor in the proximal end of the tibia. J Bone Joint Surg Am 1994;76A:549–54.

28. Brien EW, Terek RM, Healey JH, et al. Allograft reconstruction after proximal tibial resection for bone tumors. An analysis of function and outcome comparing allograft and prosthetic reconstructions. Clin Orthop 1994;303:116–27.

29. Hornicek FJ, Mnaymneh W, Lackman MD, et al. Limb salvage with osteoarticular allografts after resection of proximal tibia bone tumors. Clin Orthop 1998;352:179–85.

30. Muscolo DL, Ayerza MA, Farfalli G, et al. Proximal tibia osteoarticular allografts in tumor limb salvage surgery. Clin Orthop Relat Res 2010;468(5):1396–404.

31. Gebhardt MC, Roth YF, Mankin HJ. Osteoarticular allografts for reconstruction in the proximal part of the humerus after excision of a musculoskeletal tumor. J Bone Joint Surg Am 1990;72A:334–45.

32. Getty PJ, Peabody TD. Complications and functional outcomes of reconstruction with an osteoarticular allograft after intra-articular resection of the proximal aspect of the humerus. J Bone Joint Surg Am 1999;81A:1138–46.

33. DeGroot H, Donati D, Di Liddo M, et al. The use of cement in osteoarticular allografts for proximal humeral bone tumors. Clin Orthop 2004;427:190–7.

34. van de Sande MA, Dijkstra PD, Taminiau AH. Proximal humerus reconstruction after tumour resection: biological versus endoprosthetic reconstruction. Int Orthop 2011;35(9):1375–80.

35. Aponte-Tinao LA, Ayerza MA, Muscolo DL, et al. Allograft reconstruction for the treatment of musculoskeletal tumors of the upper extremity. Sarcoma 2013;2013:925413.

36. Kocher MS, Gebhardt MC, Manhin HJ. Reconstruction of the distal aspect of the radius with use of an osteoarticular allograft after excision of a skeletal tumor. J Bone Joint Surg Am 1998;80A:407–19.

37. Bianchi G, Donati D, Staals EL, et al. Osteoarticular allograft reconstruction of the distal radius after bone tumour resection. J Hand Surg Br 2005;30(4):369–73.

38. Scoccianti G, Campanacci DA, Beltrami G, et al. The use of osteo-articular allografts for reconstruction after resection of the distal radius for tumour. J Bone Joint Surg Br 2010;92(12):1690–4.

39. Bianchi G, Staals EL, Donati D, et al. The use of unicondylarosteoarticular allografts in reconstructions around the knee. Knee 2009;16(1):1–5.

40. Muscolo DL, Ayerza MA, Aponte-Tinao LA, et al. Unicondylarosteoarticular allografts of the knee. J Bone Joint Surg Am 2007;89(10):2137–42.

41. Fan H, Guo Z, Wang Z, et al. Surgical technique: unicondylarosteoallograft prosthesis composite in tumor limb salvage surgery. Clin Orthop Relat Res 2012;470(12):3577–86.

42. Benevenia J, Makley JT, Locke M, et al. Resection arthrodesis of the knee for tumor: large intercalary allograft and long intramedullary nail technique. Semin Arthroplasty 1994;5(2):76–84.

43. Weiner SD, Scarborough M, Vander Griend RA. Resection arthrodesis of the knee with an intercalary allograft. J Bone Joint Surg Am 1996;78A:185–92.

44. Donati D, Giacomini S, Gozzi E, et al. Allograft arthrodesis treatment of bone tumors: a two-center study. Clin Orthop 2002;400:217–24.

45. Farfalli GL, Aponte-Tinao L, Lopez-Millán L, et al. Clinical and functional outcomes of tibial intercalary allografts after tumor resection. Orthopedics 2012;35(3):e391–6.

46. Ortiz-Cruz EJ, Gebhardt MC, Jennings LC, et al. The results of transplantation of intercalary allografts after resection of tumors: a long-term follow-up study. J Bone Joint Surg Am 1997;79A:97–106.

47. Cara JA, Laclériga A, Cañadell J. Intercalary bone allografts: 23 tumor cases followed for 3 years. Acta Orthop Scand 1994;65:42–6.

48. Amitani A, Yamazaki T, Sonoda J, et al. Preservation of the knee joint in limb salvage of osteosarcoma in the proximal tibia. Int Orthop 1998;22:330–4.

49. Canadell J, Forriol F, Cara JA. Removal of metaphyseal bone tumors with preservation of the epiphysis. Physeal distraction before excision. J Bone Joint Surg Am 1994;76B:127–32.

50. Kumta SM, Chow TC, Griffith J, et al. Classifying the location of osteosarcoma with reference to the epiphyseal plate helps determine the optimal skeletal resection in limb salvage procedure. Arch Orthop Trauma Surg 1999;119:327–31.

51. Manfrini M, Gasbarrini A, Malaguti C, et al. Intraepiphyseal resection of the proximal tibia and its impact on lower limb growth. Clin Orthop 1999; 358:111–9.

52. Muscolo DL, Ayerza MA, Aponte-Tinao LA, et al. Partial epiphyseal preservation and intercalary allograft reconstruction in high-grade metaphyseal osteosarcoma of the knee. J Bone Joint Surg Am 2004;86A:2686–93.

53. Shinoara N, Sumida S, Masuda S. Bone allografts after segmental resection of tumors. Int Orthop 1990;14:273–6.

54. Tsuchiya H, Abdel-Wanis ME, Sakurakichi K, et al. Osteosarcoma around the knee. Intraepiphyseal excision and biological reconstruction with distraction osteogenesis. J Bone Joint Surg Br 2002;84B: 1162–6.

55. Li J, Wang Z, Guo Z, et al. Irregular osteotomy in limb salvage for juxta-articular osteosarcoma under computer-assisted navigation. J Surg Oncol 2012;106(4):411–6.

56. Wong KC, Kumta SM. Joint-preserving tumor resection and reconstruction using image-guided computer navigation. Clin Orthop Relat Res 2013; 471(3):762–73.

57. Deijkers RL, Bloem RM, Hogendoorn PC, et al. Hemicortical allograft reconstruction after resection of low-grade malignant bone tumours. J Bone Joint Surg Br 2002;84B:1009–14.

58. Agarwal M, Puri A, Anchan C, et al. Hemicortical excision for low-grade selected surface sarcomas of bone. Clin Orthop Relat Res 2007; 459:161–6.

59. Ayerza MA, Aponte-Tinao LA, Muscolo DL, et al. Morselized and structural cortical allograft reconstruction after intralesional curettage of a distal femoral giant-cell tumor. Orthopedics 2006;29(8): 679–82.

60. Ayerza MA, Aponte-Tinao LA, Farfalli GL, et al. Joint preservation after extensive curettage of knee giant cell tumors. Clin Orthop Relat Res 2009;467(11):2845–51.

61. Gerbers JG, Ooijen PM, Jutte PC. Computer-assisted surgery for allograft shaping in hemicortical resection: a technical note involving 4 cases. Acta Orthop 2013;84(2):224–6.

62. Aponte-Tinao LA, Ritacco LE, Ayerza MA, et al. Multiplanar osteotomies guided by navigation in chondrosarcoma of the knee. Orthopedics 2013; 36(3):e325–30.

63. Avedian RS, Haydon RC, Peabody TD. Multiplanar osteotomy with limited wide margins: a tissue preserving surgical technique for high-grade bone sarcomas. Clin Orthop Relat Res 2010;468(10): 2754–64.

64. Chen WM, Wu PK, Chen CF, et al. High-grade osteosarcoma treated with hemicortical resection and biological reconstruction. J Surg Oncol 2012; 105(8):825–9.

65. Gitelis S, Piasecki P. Allograft prosthetic composite arthroplasty for osteosarcoma and other aggressive bone tumors. Clin Orthop 1991;270: 197–201.

66. Mayle RE Jr, Paprosky WG. Massive bone loss: allograft-prosthetic composites and beyond. J Bone Joint Surg Br 2012;94(11 Suppl A):61–4.

67. Babis GC, Sakellariou VI, O'Connor MI, et al. Proximal femoral allograft-prosthesis composites in revision hip replacement: a 12-year follow-up study. J Bone Joint Surg Br 2010;92(3): 349–55.

68. Benedetti MG, Bonatti E, Malfitano C, et al. Comparison of allograft-prosthetic composite reconstruction and modular prosthetic replacement in proximal femur bone tumors: functional assessment by gait analysis in 20 patients. Acta Orthop 2013;84(2):218–23.

69. Farid Y, Lin PP, Lewis VO, et al. Endoprosthetic and allograft-prosthetic composite reconstruction of the proximal femur for bone neoplasms. Clin Orthop Relat Res 2006;442:223–9.

70. Zehr RJ, Enneking WF, Scarborough MT. Allograft-prosthesis composite versus megaprosthesis in proximal femoral reconstruction. Clin Orthop 1996;322:207–23.

71. Langlais F, Lambotte JC, Collin P, et al. Long-term results of allograft composite total hip prostheses for tumors. Clin Orthop 2003;414:197–211.

72. Muscolo DL, Farfalli GL, Aponte-Tinao LA, et al. Proximal femur allograft-prosthesis with compression plates and a short stem. Clin Orthop Relat Res 2010;468(1):224–30.

73. Biau DJ, Larousserie F, Thévenin F, et al. Results of 32 allograft-prosthesis composite reconstructions of the proximal femur. Clin Orthop Relat Res 2010;468(3):834–45.

74. Farfalli GL, Aponte-Tinao LA, Ayerza MA, et al. Comparison between constrained and semiconstrained knee allograft-prosthesis composite reconstructions. Sarcoma 2013;2013:489652. http://dx.doi.org/10.1155/2013/489652.

75. Gilbert NF, Yasko AW, Oates SD, et al. Allograft-prosthetic composite reconstruction of the proximal part of the tibia. An analysis of the early results. J Bone Joint Surg Am 2009;91(7): 1646–56.

76. Donati D, Colangeli M, Colangeli S, et al. Allograft-prosthetic composite in the proximal tibia after bone tumor resection. Clin Orthop Relat Res 2008;466(2):459–65.

77. Biau DJ, Dumaine V, Babinet A, et al. Allograft-prosthesis composites after bone tumor resection at the proximal tibia. Clin Orthop Relat Res 2007; 456:211–7.

78. Abdeen A, Hoang BH, Athanasian EA, et al. Allograft-prosthesis composite reconstruction of the proximal part of the humerus: functional outcome and survivorship. J Bone Joint Surg Am 2009;91(10):2406–15.

79. Chacon A, Virani N, Shannon R, et al. Revision arthroplasty with use of a reverse shoulder prosthesis-allograft composite. J Bone Joint Surg Am 2009;91(1):119–27.

Index

Note: Page numbers of article titles are in **boldface** type.

A

Acromioplasty
  in rotator cuff repair, **219–224**
    arthroscopic, 221–222
    introduction, 219–220
    for subacromial impingement syndrome, 220–221
Allograft(s)
  fresh frozen
    in bone and joint reconstruction, **257–269**. *See also specific allografts and* Fresh frozen allografts, in bone and joint reconstruction
Allograft-prosthetic composites
  in bone and joint reconstruction, 263–265
Anteroposterior axis
  identification of
    in measured resection technique, 178
Arthroplasty
  total knee. *See* Total knee arthroplasty (TKA)
Arthroplasty-related pseudotumor
  mimicking sarcoma, 253–254

B

Balance
  achieving of, 176–177
  defined, 158–159
Balancing techniques
  traditional, 177
Biologic agents
  in osteoporosis management, 241
Bisphosphonates
  in osteoporosis management, 240
Bone(s)
  reconstruction of
    fresh frozen allografts in, **257–269**. *See also specific allografts and* Fresh frozen allografts, in bone and joint reconstruction
Brachial plexus birth palsy, **225–232**
  anatomy related to, 225–226
  classification of, 227
  diagnosis of, 226–227
    assessment tools in, 226–227
  introduction, 225
  prevalence of, 225
  treatment of
    nonsurgical, 227
    surgical, 227–231
      microsurgery, 227–230
      osteotomies, 230–231
      tendon transfers, 230

C

Calcitonin
  in osteoporosis management, 241
Calcium supplements
  in osteoporosis management, 237–240
Circular external fixation
  in tibial fracture management, **191–206**
    case example, 200–202
    clinical results of, 197–200
      diaphyseal/segmental, 198–199
      pilon, 199–200
      plateau, 197–198
    discussion, 202–204
    half pins *vs.* wires in, 196–197
    introduction, 191–193
    vs. internal fixation methods
      indications for, 195–196
    vs. uniplanar fixation
      biomechanics of, 193–195
Coronal plane imbalance
  dynamic soft tissue balancing for, 160–161
Cyst(s)
  ganglion
    mimicking sarcoma, 248

D

Diabetic myonecrosis
  mimicking sarcoma, 251–252

E

eLibra Dynamic Knee Balancing system
  design rationale for, 179–181
  early clinical results with, 183
  surgical technique, 181–182
  troubleshooting with, 182
External fixation
  in fracture management
    history of, 191–193

F

Femoral coordinate system registration
  in TKA, 169
Force sensor
  soft tissue balance in TKA with, **175–184**. *See also* Total knee arthroplasty (TKA), soft tissue balance in, with force sensor

Orthop Clin N Am 45 (2014) 271–274
http://dx.doi.org/10.1016/S0030-5898(14)00013-3
0030-5898/14/$ – see front matter © 2014 Elsevier Inc. All rights reserved.

Moving?

Make sure your subscription moves with you!

To notify us of your new address, find your **Clinics Account Number** (located on your mailing label above your name), and contact customer service at:

Email: journalscustomerservice-usa@elsevier.com

800-654-2452 (subscribers in the U.S. & Canada)
314-447-8871 (subscribers outside of the U.S. & Canada)

Fax number: 314-447-8029

Elsevier Health Sciences Division
Subscription Customer Service
3251 Riverport Lane
Maryland Heights, MO 63043

*To ensure uninterrupted delivery of your subscription, please notify us at least 4 weeks in advance of move.